Basic Keto Recipes and Meal Planning For Beginners

70 Simple Keto Recipes and a 21-day Keto Meal Plan to Get You Started

May Green

Contents

Introduction 7
    How to Follow the Keto Diet 8
    Entering and Staying in Ketosis 11
    What Can You Eat on Keto? 12

Keto Recipes 14

Breakfast Recipes 14
    Nutty Creamy Pancakes 14
    Cauliflower and Meat Breakfast Skillet 16
    Baked Eggs in an Avocado Hole 18
    Cauliflower Cheddar Fritters 20
    Keto Hash Browns 22
    Omelet Bell Peppers 24
    Keto Breakfast Burrito 26
    Italian Eggs 28
    Sweet Potato with a Poached Egg 30
    Mushroom and Feta Keto Quiche 32
    Keto Morning Pizza 34
    Keto Muffins 36
    Keto Waffles 38
    Keto Yummy Omelet 40
    Keto Spicy Yam Breakfast Scramble 42
    Keto Sausage and Pepper Breakfast Casserole ... 44
    Keto Cinnamon Rolls 46
    Keto Breakfast Chia Pudding 50
    Keto Oatmeal with Berries 52
    Keto Breakfast Bake 54

Lunch Recipes 56
    Taco Stuffed Avocados 56

Bacon Sushi 58
Keto Shrimp Lettuce Wraps.. 60
Keto Egg and Cucumber Salad 62
Salmon Wrapped with Prosciutto 63
Burger Bombs 64
Cauliflower Nachos 66
Zucchini Pasta Salad 68
Keto Quesadilla 70
Keto Grilled Cheese Sandwich 72
Stuffed Tomato Cheeseburgers 74
Turkey Cheese Keto Roll-Ups.. 76
Keto Stuffed Poblano Peppers... 78
Italian Keto Roll-Ups 80

Dinner Recipes 82
Oven Baked Chicken with Garlic 82
Salmon with Lemon 84
Keto Bacon-Wrapped Meatloaf.. 86
Low-Carb Lamb Sliders 88
Keto Cuban Roast Pork 90
Keto Chicken Wings 92
Keto Bacon Cheeseburger Bake 94
Tuna Casserole 96
Keto Stuffed Bell Peppers.. 98
Keto Pesto Salmon.. 100
Pimiento Cheese Meatballs with Zucchini Pasta 102
Roasted Turkey with Keto Cream Cheese Sauce....................... 104
Keto Crack Chicken 106
Keto Chicken Enchilada 108

Ketogenic Soups 110
Keto Chili.. 110
Keto Cream of Asparagus 112

Keto Cauliflower Bacon Chowder 114

Keto Thai Curry Soup 116

Keto Cream of Zucchini 118

Ketogenic Desserts 120

Coconut Macadamia Bars 120

Almond Butter Pie 122

Flourless Chocolate Brownies 124

No-Bake Peanut Butter Chocolate Bars 126

Keto Peppermint Bars 128

Keto Carrot Cake 130

Keto No-Bake Coconut Peanut Butter Cookies 132

Carb-Free Raspberry Dream Cheesecake 134

Keto Chocolate Mug Cake 136

Salted Caramel Cake Bombs 138

Chocolate Blueberry Clusters Keto 140

Keto Lemon Bars 142

Ketogenic Sauces & Dressings 144

Keto Ranch 144

Keto Honey Mustard 146

Keto Ketchup 148

Keto Hollandaise 150

Keto BBQ Sauce 152

21-DAY KETO MEAL PLAN 154

Day 1 154

Day 2 154

Day 3 154

Day 4 155

Day 5 155

Day 6 155

Day 7 156

Day 8 156
Day 9 156
Day 10 157
Day 11 157
Day 12 157
Day 13 158
Day 14 158
Day 15 158
Day 16 159
Day 17 159
Day 18 159
Day 19 160
Day 20 160
Day 21 160

Text Copyright © May Green

All rights reserved. No part of this guide may be reproduced in any form without permission in writing from the publisher except in the case of brief quotations embodied in critical articles or reviews.

Introduction

Welcome to our ketogenic cookbook! This cookbook is about to change your life for the better. You will enter a world of new eating habits, which will bring about weight loss and health galore.

First of all, it is wonderful that you have chosen this book. The ketogenic diet will not disappoint you. This new way of eating is a remarkable way to turn your body into a fat-burning machine by limiting carbs and upping your intake of carbs. As your body runs out of glucose from carbs to burn for energy, it starts to burn your body fat, forming ketone bodies. Your body uses these ketone bodies for energy in place of carbs. This places you in a state of ketosis, the state in which your body starts using more ketones than glucose to fuel your body.

Ketosis leads to significant weight loss. But it has other benefits as well. These include:

- You will feel fuller, so you don't have as many food cravings.
- You will lose weight quicker.
- You will feel more energetic.
- Your blood sugars will be more stable. Your blood pressure and cholesterol levels will stabilize too.
- Your skin will clear up.
- Your chronic pain will decrease.
- You will have less seizures if you're epileptic.
- You will have fewer joint problems.
- You will be able to enjoy many keto version of your favorite foods … without any guilt!

How to Follow the Keto Diet

The ketogenic diet uses very low carbs and very high fat to make your body enter the state of ketosis. When you eat lots of carbohydrates and sugar, they are more readily converted to glucose, your body's preferred fuel source. As a result of the ready availability of glucose, your body does not burn its stores of body fat for fuel. When carbohydrates and sugar are no longer readily available, your body is forced to burn its stores of fat. This makes you lose weight!

Another benefit of the ketogenic diet is that you do not eat sugar, which has been associated with inflammation. This makes the ketogenic diet if you suffer from pain related to endometriosis, neuropathy, fibromyalgia, arthritis, and other pain-related medical issues. Furthermore, the lack of sugar is also beneficial if you suffer from diabetes, heart disease, and stomach problems. Last but not the least, as the ketogenic diet was originally invented as way to treat epilepsy, it is a great diet to follow if you suffer from seizures or neurological disorders such as Alzheimer's disease and Parkinson's disease.

The ketogenic diet, aka "keto" is easy to follow once you learn the basics. However, to enjoy the benefits of keto, you cannot simply eliminate sugar. You also need to nourish your body with sufficient protein and fat, and eat some carbohydrates, since your brain cannot function without them.

Also, like with any other diet, you *will* gain weight if you overeat. You must keep your daily calories under a certain limit to maintain or lose weight.

Here is the way to figure out the amount of calories that you need to consume each day. First of all, you figure out how many calories you need to consume in order to maintain your weight, and then you figure out how many calories you need to consume to lose weight. Next, you break your caloric requirements down into macronutrients to figure out how much carbohydrate, protein, and fat you need to consume each day.

Step 1: Find your BMR value, or basal metabolic rate.

For men, 66 + (6.3 x body weight in pounds) + (12.9 x height in inches) + (6.8 x age in years) = BMR

For women, 655 + (4.3 x body weight in pounds) + (4.7 x height in inches) + (4.7 x age in years) = BMR

Step 2: Find the daily caloric requirements needed to maintain your current body weight.

If you are sedentary (no activity): BMR x 1.2

If you are lightly active (exercise 1-3 hours a week): BMR x 1.375

If you are moderately active (exercise 3-5 hours a week): BMR x 1.55

If you are very active (exercise 6-7 hours per week): BMR x 1.725

If you are extremely active (such as an athlete or practice extreme sports): BMR x 1.9

Step 3: Find the daily caloric requirements to lose weight.

There are 3,500 calories in a pound of fat. To lose weight, decrease your daily caloric requirements by 500. Then you can reasonably expect to lose 1 pound in seven days.

Step 4: Find your macros. This depends on your particular keto diet. Using classic keto as an example, you should consume 40 to 70% of your daily caloric requirement as fat, 15

to 30% of your daily caloric requirement as protein, and 15 to 30% of your daily requirement as carbs. So, if your daily caloric requirements are 2000 calories and you want to lose 1 pound per week, you will need to consume 1500 calories a day.

Use this formula to calculate your macros:

For protein: 1500 x .3 = 450 calories from protein

For carbs: 1500 x .15 = 225 calories from carbs

For fat: 1500 x .55 = 825 calories from fat

Step 5: Break down the calories into grams. Now you have your macros. However, calories are often not split into macros on food labels. That is why breaking calories down further into grams per macronutrient is helpful.

Fat has 9 calories per gram. Divide the calories from fat by 9 to get the grams from fat.

Protein has 4 calories per gram. Divide the calories from protein by 4 to get the grams from protein.

Carbohydrates have 4 calories per gram. Divide the calories from carbs by 4 to get the grams from carbs.

On a classic keto diet, following a 2000-calorie diet, you will need 83-125 grams of fat per day, under 20 grams of carb per day, and somewhere around 20-40 grams of protein per day. But you will need to adjust these numbers for your unique daily caloric requirements found in Steps 2 and 3. However, there are many different forms of keto that specify different macro ratios. Be sure to get familiar with the specific macro requirements of your particular keto diet.

Entering and Staying in Ketosis

The keto diet only leads to weight loss when you are in the state of ketosis. Usually, it takes up to five days of not eating carbs to enter ketosis. To confirm that you are in ketosis, you can perform urine ketone tests, which are available at major retailers such as Amazon and Walmart. Only when the test reads that you have ketone levels at or above 1.0 are you truly in ketosis.

You should test your ketone level daily. If your readings fall below 1.0, you are no longer in ketosis. You may fall out of ketosis if you are eating too many carbs, too many grams of protein, or if you enjoyed a cheat meal. While being out of ketosis for a few hours is OK every now and then, being out of ketosis for too long will stall or reverse your weight loss and health benefits. To get back into ketosis, you need to decrease your carb intake or engage in a 48-hour water fast to get back on track.

What Can You Eat on Keto?

This book is full of great keto recipes. You can find many more online. This diet is hardly restrictive; you can find all sorts of delicious goodies that are low-carb or carb-free. If you are craving brownies, for instance, you can find recipes for keto-friendly brownies!

What food can you eat? You can eat all sorts of foods on keto. However, foods that are carb-free or low on the glycemic index are great. No, you can't eat regular white bread and non-keto pasta and non-keto cakes on this diet. However, instead of focusing on what you can't eat, think about all that you *can* eat. Keto lets you enjoy a wide range of delicious foods! These include:

- Berries
- Meat
- Cheese
- Cottage cheese
- Avocados
- Salad greens
- Oil and vinegar on salads
- Seeds
- Low-carb nuts like almonds
- Eggs
- Kefir
- Non-starchy vegetables
- Fish
- Coconut flour
- Almond flour
- Almond or cashew or coconut milk

This cookbook includes inspiring and delicious ketogenic recipes using ingredients you can find in any grocery store.

These recipes taste great and replace the high-carb treats you are used to eating. There is also a meal plan to help you launch your journey into ketosis!

So, let's not waste a second. It's time to launch your ketogenic journey and start losing weight and enjoying better health!

Keto Recipes

To jumpstart your keto diet, here are 70 delicious recipes that you will love. These recipes are stunningly low in carbs and high in fat! Following these recipes is a 21-day meal plan which uses some of the recipes.

Breakfast Recipes

Nutty Creamy Pancakes

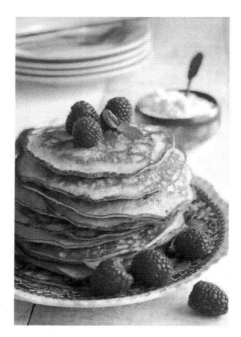

Ingredients

- 4 oz cream cheese
- 4 eggs
- 3 tbsp almond flour
- pinch salt
- Butter

Directions

1. Blend all ingredients in a blender.
2. Butter griddle.
3. Pour batter on the griddle. Cook for 1 minute on each side.
4. Serve with berries, lox with cream cheese, peanut butter, or bacon and cheese.

Nutritional Information

Servings: 4 pancakes
Calories: 52 per pancake
Fat: 5 g
Protein: 2 g
Carbs: 3 g

Cauliflower and Meat Breakfast Skillet

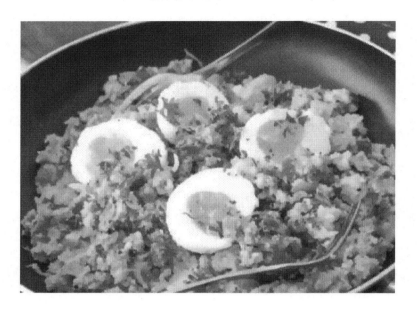

Ingredients

- 4 bacon strips
- 4 eggs, boiled
- 2 cs. cauliflower blended into fine chunks
- 1/2 onion, diced
- 1/2 red bell pepper, diced
- 1/2 c heavy whipping cream
- 1/2 tsp paprika
- 1 tbsp butter
- Salt and pepper to taste

Directions

1. Sauté onion and bacon until soft and cooked through.
2. Mix in cauliflower, red bell pepper, paprika, butter, salt, and pepper.
3. Sauté mixture for 5-10 minutes.
4. Stir in heavy cream until everything is bubbling and well mixed.
5. Garnish with eggs and parsley if you wish.
6. Serve hot and enjoy!

Nutritional Information

Servings: 4 cups
Calories: 130 per cup
Fat: 10 g
Protein: 6 g
Carbs: 1 g

Baked Eggs in an Avocado Hole

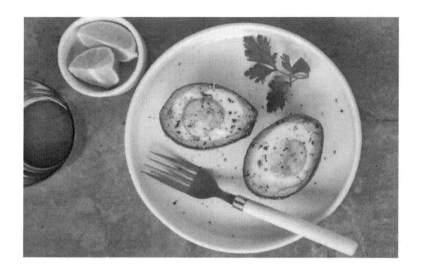

Ingredients

- 1 large avocado
- 2 eggs
- Salt and pepper to taste
- Chives
- 1 tsp paprika
- 1 tbsp parmesan cheese

Directions

1. Slice avocado in half. Spoon out to make hole bigger.
2. Crack eggs, placing one egg into each avocado half.
3. Top with parmesan cheese and paprika.
4. Line outside of each halved avocado with foil.
5. Bake for 15 minutes at 425°F.

Nutritional Information

Servings: 1 baked avocado
Calories: 472 per avocado
Fat: 34 g
Protein: 18 g
Carbs: 17 g

Cauliflower Cheddar Fritters

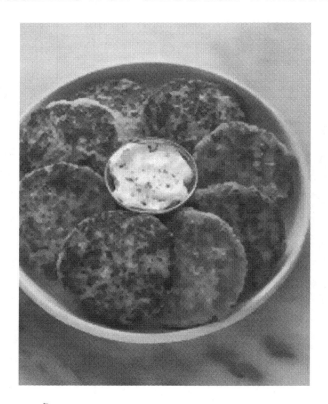

Ingredients

- 1 tbsp finely ground flaxseed
- 3 tbsps butter
- Cauliflower, half head blended to meal
- ½ c scallions, sliced
- 3 tbsp. cheddar cheese, finely grated
- 2 eggs
- 1 ½ tsp salt
- ½ tsp pepper
- 3 tbsps sour cream, to serve

Directions

1. Combine cauliflower and salt in a bowl. Use some cheesecloth to wring some moisture from the cauliflower.
2. Add all the ingredients except the butter and sour cream to the cauliflower.
3. Melt butter and add to mixture.
4. Spoon mixture onto the pan in small heaps and flatten with the back of a spoon or spatula.
5. Fry until golden brown. Serve with sour cream and chives.

Nutritional Information

Servings: 8 fritters
Calories: 225 per 2 fritters
Fat: 18 g
Protein: 8 g
Carbs: 8 g

Keto Hash Browns

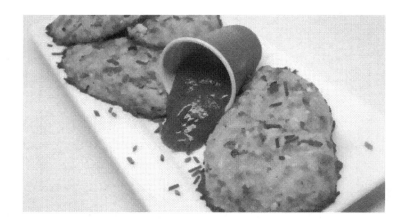

Ingredients

- 3 cs cauliflower, processed into meal
- 1 c cheddar cheese, shredded
- 1 egg
- ¼ c bacon, crumbled
- ½ tsp salt
- 1/8 tsp black pepper
- Cayenne pepper if you want it spicy
- 1 tbsp diced chives

Directions

1. Preheat oven to 400°F.
2. Microwave cauliflower. Pat with a towel to remove some moisture.
3. Mix all ingredients in a bowl. Spoon onto a baking sheet and divide into 6 servings.
4. Bake for 15 minutes at 400°F. Broil for 5 minutes to get crispy.
5. Serve with keto ketchup or other sauce of your choice.

Nutritional Information

Servings: 6 hashbrowns
Calories: 118 per hashbrown
Fat: 8.2 g
Protein: 8.8 g
Carbs: 3 g

Omelet Bell Peppers

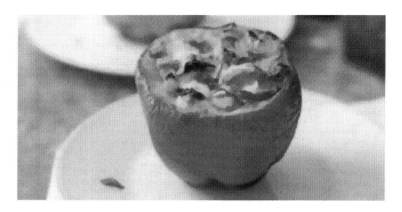

Ingredients

- 2 bell peppers, gutted (orange is medium, yellow savory, red sweet)
- 8 eggs, whisked
- 1 c cheddar cheese, shredded
- ¼ c whole milk (more fat is best!)
- 4 slices crispy bacon, broken up
- 2 tbsp chives
- Salt and pepper to taste
- Hot sauce to taste

Directions

1. Bake peppers at 400°F with a little water inside. Wrap foil outside to prevent burning.
2. Mix all other ingredients in a bowl. Pour inside peppers when they are done baking.
3. Wrap peppers in foil and bake for 35-40 minutes at 400°F or until eggs harden.

Nutritional Information

Servings: 2 peppers
Calories: 209 per pepper
Fat: 24 g
Protein: 29 g
Carbs: 3 g

Keto Breakfast Burrito

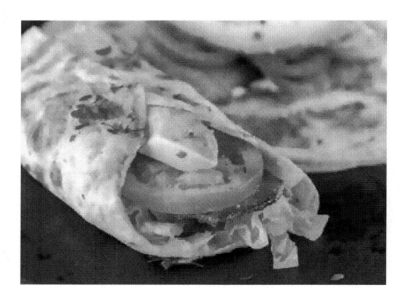

Ingredients

- 2 eggs
- 1/4 tsp dried coriander
- 1/4 tsp dried cumin
- 1 tbsp rosemary, freshly chopped
- 1 tsp onion flakes
- pinch chili powder
- 1/4 c cheese, grated or shredded
- 1 tsp dried garlic
- 1 tsp poppy seeds
- 1 tbsp chopped chives
- 1 tbsp butter
- 2 tbsp heavy cream

Directions

1. Whisk everything but the butter.
2. Melt butter in a pan. Add egg mixture and let cook until firm.
3. Place a lid over the pan and let burrito cook for 2 minutes.
4. Add whatever fillings you wish ... sausage, eggs, cheese, jalapenos, tomatoes, and avocado.
5. Roll up and top with cheese and chili powder if you wish. Dip with sour cream or keto ranch.

Nutritional Information

Servings: 1 burrito
Calories: 331 per burrito
Fat: 30 g
Protein: 11 g
Carbs: 1 g

Italian Eggs

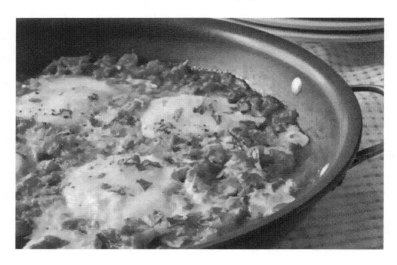

Ingredients

- 1/2 c spinach, chopped
- 1/2 c marinara sauce
- 2 eggs
- 1/4 c mozzarella cheese, shredded
- Salt and pepper to taste

Directions

1. Heat marinara in a small pan and mix with spinach and eggs. Season. Top with cheese
2. Heat till bubbling. Then cover and simmer for 3 minutes for soft boiled eggs or 5 minutes for hard boiled.

Nutritional Information

Servings: 1 cup
Calories: 200 per cup
Fat: 15 g
Protein: 13 g
Carbs: 3 g

Sweet Potato with a Poached Egg

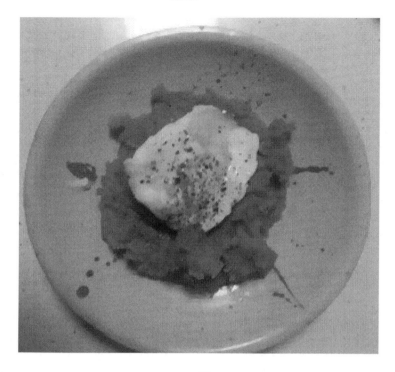

Ingredients

- butter
- 1 sweet potato
- 2 eggs
- 4 crispy strips bacon, crumbled
- Basil, chopped

Directions

1. Melt butter.
2. Peel then grate the sweet potato. Mix into butter and cook for ten minutes on the stove until soft and mushy.
3. Boil a saucepan full of water and crack in eggs. Boil for 2 minutes until poached.
4. Put sweet potato on plate then add eggs and crumbled bacon on top.
5. Add cheese or seasonings or parsley to garnish if you like.

Nutritional Information

Servings: 1
Calories: 264 for 1 serving
Fat: 5.1 g
Protein: 9.1 g
Carbs: 27 g

Mushroom and Feta Keto Quiche

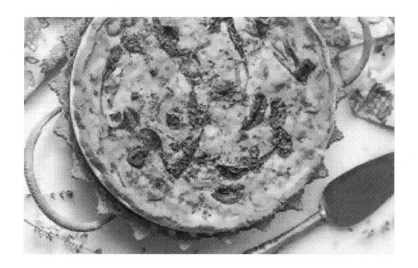

Ingredients

- 8 oz button mushrooms
- 1 clove garlic
- 10 oz box frozen spinach, thawed
- 4 large eggs
- 1 c milk
- 2 oz feta cheese
- 1/4 c parmesan powder
- 1/2 c mozzarella cheese, shredded

Directions

1. Preheat oven to 350°F.
2. Thaw spinach and wring out moisture. Mince garlic. Wash veggies.
3. Put mushrooms, garlic, and salt in a skillet. Sauté until soft and mushrooms brown.
4. Place spinach in dish and put mushrooms on top. Top with feta cheese.
5. Whisk eggs with milk and parmesan powder. Add pepper if you wish. Pour over veggie and cheese mixture. Sprinkle mozzarella on top.
6. Bake for 45-55 minutes. Slice and serve warm.

Nutritional Information

Servings: 6 slices
Calories: 481 per slice
Fat: 38 g
Protein: 17 g
Carbs: 20 g

Keto Morning Pizza

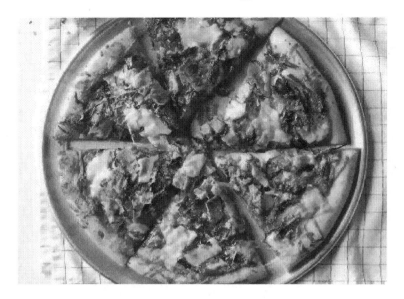

Ingredients

- Olive oil
- 4 eggs
- 2 tbsps water
- 1 tsp garlic powder
- 1 tsp onion powder
- 1 tsp dried oregano
- ¼ c coconut flour
- 6 tbsps parmesan cheese, grated
- 1 c spinach leaves
- 2 bell peppers, thinly sliced
- 6 bacon strips
- 1 c provolone cheese, shredded
- 6 eggs

Directions

1. Preheat oven to 400°F. Line two pans with parchment paper and spray with olive oil.
2. Cook bacon until crisp, then drain. Crumble bacon.
3. Whisk eggs with water, garlic powder, onion powder, and oregano powder.
4. Stir flour into eggs and beating, remove lumps. Add parmesan cheese.
5. Thicken by resting. Then transfer into pans. Spread out evenly.
6. Bake for 10 minutes.
7. Remove crusts. Spritz with oil. Place half of the shredded provolone cheese onto the crust with spinach leaves and peppers.
8. Break eggs and then slide them onto pizza.
9. Bake until egg whites are set.
10. Sprinkle more bacon on top.
11. Cool and then slice.

Nutritional Information

Servings: 6 slices
Calories: 544 per slice
Fat: 38 g
Protein: 38 g
Carbs: 9 g

Keto Muffins

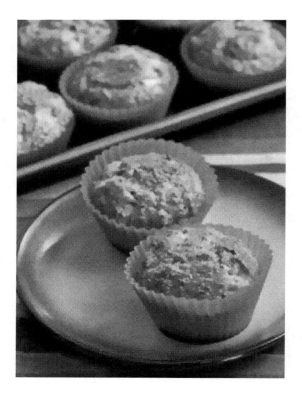

Ingredients

- 1/2 c almond flour
- 1/2 c raw hemp seeds
- 1/2 c finely grated parmesan cheese
- 1/4 c flaxseed meal
- 1/4 c nutritional yeast flakes
- 1/2 tsp baking powder
- 1/2 tsp seasoning salt
- 1/3 c green onion, thinly sliced
- 1/4 tsp salt
- 6 eggs, beaten
- ½ c cottage cheese

Directions

1. Preheat oven to 375°F. Oil muffin pan.
2. Mix flour, hemp seed, cheese, flaxseed, yeast, baking powder, and seasonings.
3. Beat eggs and add cottage cheese and onions.
4. Mix wet and dry ingredients together.
5. Fill muffin cups with mixture.
6. Bake for 25-30 minutes. Serve warm with butter and liquid keto sweetener (e.g. liquid stevia).

Nutritional Information

Servings: 6 muffins
Calories: 230 per muffin
Fat: 20 g
Protein: 5 g
Carbs: 3 g

Keto Waffles

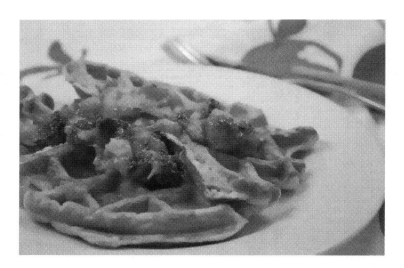

Ingredients

- 3 egg whites
- 2 tbsps coconut flour
- 2 tbsps milk
- 1/2 tsp baking powder
- Keto sweetener to taste (e.g. stevia)

Directions

1. Whisk eggs into stiff peaks.
2. Add flour, milk, baking powder, keto sweetener, and egg.
3. Heat up waffle iron. Pour on batter. Cook until browned.
4. Serve with butter, keto-friendly sugar-free syrup, cheese and bacon, or sugar-free jam.

Nutritional Information

Servings: 1
Calories: 121 per waffle
Fat: 1 g
Protein: 20 g
Carbs: 2.1 g

Keto Yummy Omelet

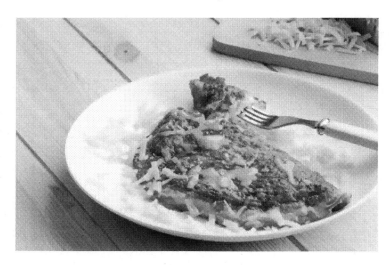

Ingredients

- 6 eggs
- 2 tbsps sour cream
- Salt and pepper to taste
- 3 oz cheese, shredded, divided
- 2 oz butter
- 5 oz diced deli ham
- ½ yellow onion
- ½ green bell pepper

Directions

1. In a mixing bowl, whisk eggs with cream and add salt and pepper, and half of the shredded cheese.
2. Melt the butter on medium heat.
3. Sauté ham, onion and peppers together. Add eggs. Fry until almost firm.
4. Reduce heat to low. Add cheese on top and fold in half.
5. Sauté the diced ham, onion and peppers for a few minutes. Add the egg mixture and fry until the omelet is almost firm. Be extra mindful not to burn the edges.
6. Reduce the heat after a little while. Sprinkle the rest of the cheese on top and fold omelet. Garnish with sliced green onions or chives.

Nutritional Information

Servings: 1
Calories: 256
Fat: 20 g
Protein: 14 g
Carbs: 5 g

Keto Spicy Yam Breakfast Scramble

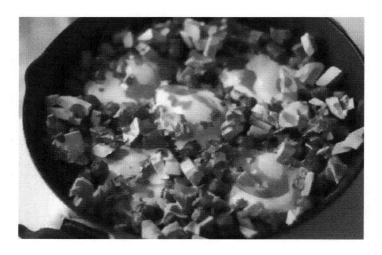

Ingredients

- 1 lb breakfast sausage
- 2 sweet potatoes, diced
- 5 eggs
- Salt and pepper to taste
- 1 avocado, diced
- Handful cilantro
- Hot sauce (optional)

Directions

1. Preheat your oven to 400°F.
2. Brown sausage. Use slotted spoon to remove sausage and drain fat.
3. Cook the sweet potatoes in the sausage grease.
4. Add sausage back into the pan.
5. Crack eggs into sausage mixture.
6. Place skillet in oven and bake for 5 minutes or until eggs harden. Broil for one minute.
7. Remove from oven and add avocado and cilantro. Add hot sauce if you wish. Add salt and pepper and serve hot.

Nutritional Information

Servings: 4 cups
Calories: 190 per cup
Fat: 12 g
Protein: 10 g
Carbs: 5 g

Keto Sausage and Pepper Breakfast Casserole

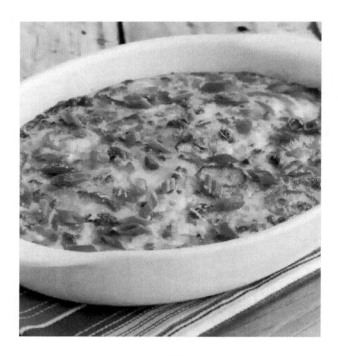

Ingredients

- 10 whole eggs
- 12 oz Italian sausage, cooked and crumbled
- 3 cs. cheddar cheese, shredded, divided
- 1/4 c onions, minced and sautéed
- 1/2 c roasted red pepper, chopped
- 1/3 c heavy cream
- 1/2 c cream cheese
- 1 tsp garlic salt
- 1/2 tsp cayenne pepper (optional)
- 2 tbsps parsley, dried

Directions

1. Preheat oven to 350°F.
2. Whisk eggs, spices and heavy cream together in bowl.
3. Pour half of the egg mixture into a baking dish.
4. Add sausage, peppers, cheese, and onions to the egg mixture from step 3.
5. Dollop cream choose on top of the sausage mixture.
6. Add the rest of the egg mixture.
7. Sprinkle with shredded cheddar cheese.
8. Bake for 30 minutes or until toothpick comes out clean.
9. Cool then cut into pieces.

Nutritional Information

Servings: 6 cups
Calories: 424 per cup
Fat: 33 g
Protein: 24 g
Carbs: 5 g

Keto Cinnamon Rolls

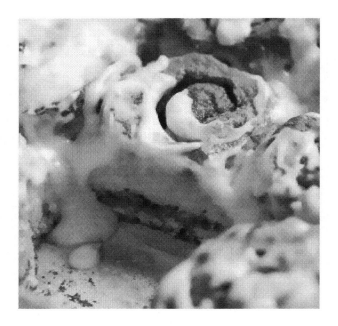

Ingredients

- 2 ¼ c flour, almond or coconut
- 2 ¼ tsp baking powder
- 1/4 c sour cream
- 2 tsp apple cider vinegar
- 3 tbsps lukewarm water
- 1 tbsp honey
- 1 tbsp active dry yeast
- ground ginger to taste
- 6 tbsp flaxseed meal
- 5 tbsps whey protein
- 4-6 tsps erythritol
- 2 ¼ tsps xanthan gum
- 2 tsp sea salt
- 3 eggs at room temperature
- 1 1/2 tbsps. coconut oil
- 1 tbsp apple cider vinegar

- 3 tbsps butter, softened
- 4-6 tbsps erythritol, to taste
- 2 tbsps cinnamon
- 1/3 c cream cheese, softened
- 3 tbsps. butter
- 3-6 tbsps. powdered erythritol
- 1 tsp vanilla extract
- pinch salt
- 2 c almond milk

Directions

1. Line small pan with parchment paper in small pan. Lay down plastic wrap on to work surface to roll dough. Have a small bowl of water with a drizzle of oil nearby.
2. Mix sour cream, water and honey in a bowl. Set over water that feels slightly warm to touch but is not boiling.
3. Add yeast and ginger. Pour sour cream mixture over yeast and cover and rest for 7 minutes until it looks bubbly.
4. While the yeast is rising, mix the flours together.
5. To the flour mixture, add flaxseed meal, whey protein powder, sweetener, xanthan gum, baking powder, and salt and thoroughly mix. Set aside.
6. When the yeast is proofed, add the eggs, melted butter and vinegar. Mix well for 1minute. Now add the flour mixture and mix thoroughly until very sticky.
7. Divide into 3 mounds and oil some cling wrap. Lay dough on it to work with. Spread each mound of dough into a rectangle, brush with melted butter, and sprinkle with cinnamon. Roll dough tightly and seal edges by pinching with your wet fingers.
8. Cut the rectangles into thirds. Press down. Now cover with a towel and leave in a warm place to rise for 1 hour.

9. Preheat oven to 400°F.
10. Make glaze by mixing together cream cheese, butter, and sweetener until fluffy. Add in the vanilla extract, salt, and milk. Set aside.
11. Now roll up dough. Place in oven and bake for 25 minutes, covered in loose foil.
12. Let cool. Spread glaze on top.

Nutritional Information

Servings: 6 rolls
Calories: 319 per roll
Fat: 29 g
Protein: 8 g
Carbs: 8 g

Keto Breakfast Chia Pudding

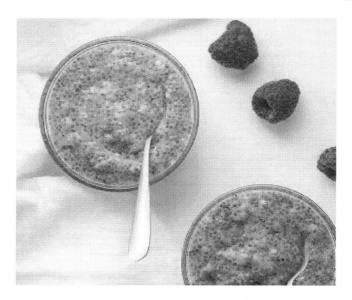

Ingredients

- 1/4 c chia seeds
- 1 c full-fat coconut milk
- 1/2 tbsp honey
- Berries of your choice

Directions

1. Mix chia seeds, coconut milk, and honey together in a small bowl or glass mason jar.
2. Let it set in refrigerator overnight.
3. Make sure the chia has gelled.
4. Garnish with berries and enjoy cold.

Nutritional Information

Servings: 2
Calories: 206 for 1 serving
Fat: 14.4 g
Protein: 4.6 g
Carbs: 20.3 g

Keto Oatmeal with Berries

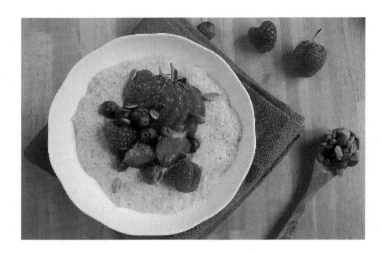

Ingredients

- 1/2 c unsweetened vanilla almond milk
- 1/4 c coconut flour
- 2 tbsp. unsweetened coconut flakes
- 1 tbsp flaxseed meal
- 1 tbsp chia seeds
- 1/2 tbsp monk fruit
- 1/2 tsp cinnamon
- pinch salt
- 1/2 tsp vanilla extract

Directions

1. Mix all the ingredients except the milk and vanilla in a pot.
2. Then add milk and vanilla and bring to a boil.
3. When it is rolling, reduce to a simmer until it thickens. This should take about 1 minute.
4. Add berries, and chopped nuts if you wish.
5. Add in the milk and vanilla and bring to a boil over high heat.

Nutritional Information

Servings: 2
Calories: 327 for 1 serving
Fat: 27. 3 g
Protein: 11 g
Carbs: 15. 6 g

Keto Breakfast Bake

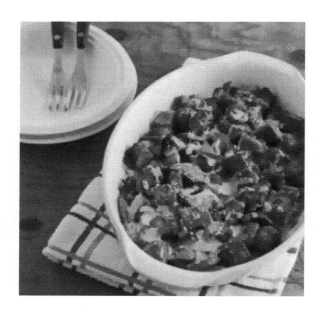

Ingredients

- 2 bell peppers of different colors
- 1 tsp olive oil
- 1/2 tsp olive oil
- Season-All and black pepper to taste
- 12 links sausage of any kind
- ½ c shredded mozzarella cheese

Directions

1. Preheat oven to 450°F. Grease baking dish.
2. Cut peppers into small pieces. Toss with 1 tsp olive oil and sprinkle with seasonings. Place in greased baking dish and place in oven for 20 minutes.
3. As they cook, heat rest of the oil in pan and cook sausages for 10-12 minutes.
4. Slice sausages. Add to peppers once they are done cooking and bake for 5 minutes.
5. Sprinkle mozzarella on top and broil for 5 minutes.
6. Serve hot with salt and pepper to taste. You can also add cayenne for a nice kick.

Nutritional Information

Servings: 3 cups
Calories: 349 per cup
Fat: 29 g
Protein: 20 g
Carbs: 5 g

Lunch Recipes
Taco Stuffed Avocados

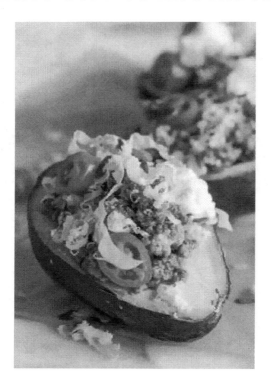

Ingredients

- 4 ripe avocados
- 1 lb hamburger
- juice of 1 lime
- 1 tbsp extra-virgin olive oil
- 1 onion, chopped
- 1 packet taco seasoning
- Black pepper and sea salt to taste
- Cheese, tomato, lettuce, guacamole, and sour cream (optional for toppings)

Directions

1. Halve and pit avocados. Spoon out more to make a bigger hole. Dice the avocado flesh that has been removed and set aside for later. Squeeze lime juice over all the avocados.
2. Heat oil in a pan and add onion and sauté until tender. Add beef, taco seasoning and salt and pepper. Cook until beef browns. Drain fat.
3. Fill avocado holes with mixture. Top with chopped avocado, lettuce, tomato, and sour cream or guacamole

Nutritional Information

Servings: 8 stuffed avocados
Calories: 150 per avocado half
Fat: 15 g
Protein: 16 g
Carbs: 5 g

Bacon Sushi

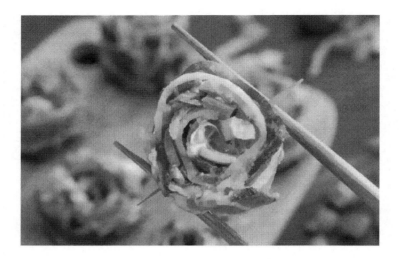

Ingredients

- 10 slices of bacon
- 2 tbsp. mayonnaise
- 1 c. tomatoes
- 1/2 avocado, diced
- 1 c. romaine lettuce, shredded
- Kosher salt
- Freshly ground black pepper

Directions

1. Preheat oven to 400°F and lay wire rack over baking sheet. Weave the ten bacon slices over each other to make a square. Bake for 20 minutes.
2. Pat with paper towel. Place on plastic wrap.
3. Add mayo to top of bacon lattice. Top bottom part of bacon with avocado and tomatoes. Place romaine lettuce on top and add salt and pepper to taste.
4. Roll tightly. Slice into 6 rolls.

Nutritional Information

Servings: 6 rolls
Calories: 130 per roll
Fat: 10 g
Protein: 5 g
Carbs: 0 g

Keto Shrimp Lettuce Wraps

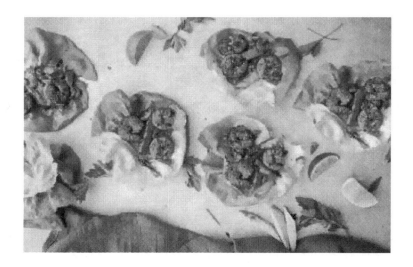

Ingredients

- 1/4 tbsp. butter
- 2 garlic cloves, minced
- 1/2 c. blue cheese, crumbled
- 1/4 c. hot sauce
- 1 tbsp. extra-virgin olive oil
- 1 lb. shrimp, peeled and tails cut off
- Kosher salt
- Black pepper, freshly ground
- 1 head romaine lettuce, leaves separated, for serving
- 1/4 red onion, chopped
- 1 celery stalk, thinly sliced

Directions

1. Melt butter and add garlic and cook until fragrant. Then add hot sauce. Simmer over low heat. This is your buffalo sauce.
2. Cook shrimp in oil with salt and pepper for 2 minutes. Add buffalo sauce and toss to coat.
3. Scoop into romaine leaf. Top with other veggies and blue cheese.

Nutritional Information

Servings: 10 wraps
Calories: 60 per wrap
Fat: 4 g
Protein: 4 g
Carbs: 1 g

Keto Egg and Cucumber Salad

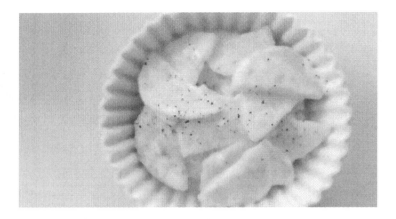

Ingredients

- 1 cucumber, sliced
- 2 tbsps lemon juice
- 2 tbsps mayonnaise
- Salt and pepper to taste

Directions

Combine cucumber, mayonnaise, and lemon juice in a salad bowl. Season with salt and pepper to taste.

Nutritional Information

Servings: 1
Calories: 117 for 1 serving
Fat: 11 g
Protein: 0.8 g
Carbs: 4.8 g

Salmon Wrapped with Prosciutto

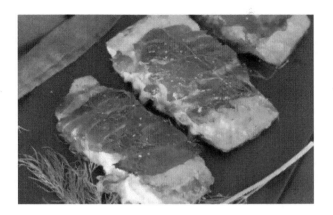

Ingredients

- 3 oz-salmon filet
- 2 thin slices prosciutto
- ½ tsp olive oil, salt and pepper to taste

Directions

1. Preheat oven to 425°F.
2. Add salt and pepper to the salmon filet and wrap in the prosciutto, leaving ends open. Place face down in an oiled pan.
3. Drizzle with 1/2 tsp oil.
4. Bake in middle of oven for 8 to 9 minutes.

Nutritional Information

Servings: 1
Calories: 179
Fat: 17 g
Protein: 10 g
Carbs: 0 g

Burger Bombs

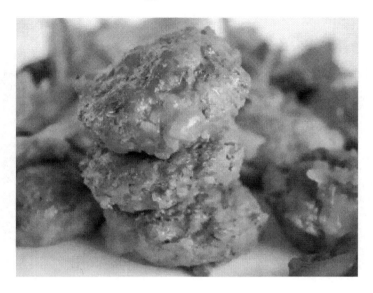

Ingredients

- 12 slices bacon
- 12 cubes cheddar cheese
- 12 sausage patties, uncooked
- Cumin, onion powder, salt and pepper to taste

Directions

1. Preheat oven to 350°F. Line a baking dish with foil. Lay out sausage patties with some space in between.
2. Add seasonings and cheddar cheese in the center of each sausage patty.
3. Squeeze sausage patties into balls so that the cheese is enclosed.
4. Wrap balls in bacon.
5. Bake for 60 minutes.
6. Serve with keto ketchup or keto ranch.

Nutritional Information

Servings: 12 bombs
Calories: 249 per bomb
Fat: 20 g
Protein: 15 g
Carbs: 1.4 g

Cauliflower Nachos

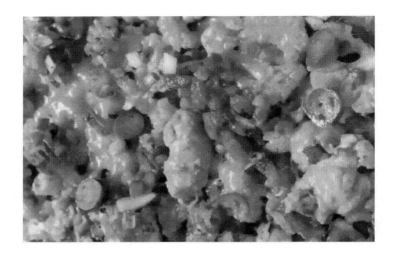

Ingredients

- 2 small heads cauliflower, chopped
- 3 tbsp extra-virgin olive oil
- 1 tsp salt
- 1/2 tsp cumin
- 1/2 tsp paprika
- 1/4 tsp chili powder
- 1/4 tsp garlic powder
- 1 c. Colby cheese, shredded

Directions

1. Preheat oven to 425°F.
2. Add cauliflower and coat in oil. Sprinkle with spices and toss. Roast for 20-25 minutes.
3. Top with Colby cheese and bake till melted (about 5 minutes).
4. Serve with salsa, jalapenos, sour cream, and guacamole if you wish.

Nutritional Information

Servings: 4 cups
Calories: 288 per cup
Fat: 21 g
Protein: 10 g
Carbs: 18g

Zucchini Pasta Salad

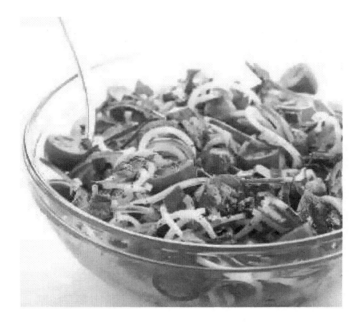

Ingredients

- 3 zucchini, spiraled
- 3 tbsp cooking oil
- 1/2 tbsp lemon juice
- 1/4 tsp garlic powder
- 1/4 tsp sea salt
- 1/8 tsp black pepper
- 6 slices bacon, crumbled
- 1 1/2 c grape tomatoes, halved
- 1 tsp rosemary

Directions

1. Whisk oil, lemon juice, and seasonings in a bowl.
2. Now combine zucchini, tomatoes, bacon, and rosemary. Toss with the oil mixture.

Nutritional Information

Servings: 4 cups
Calories: 153 per cup
Fat: 12g
Protein: 6g
Carbs: 7g

Keto Quesadilla

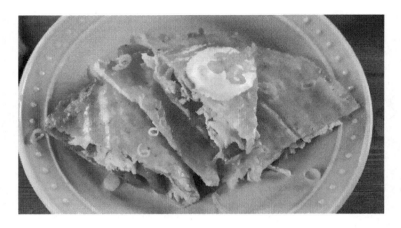

Ingredients

For Tortillas:

- 2 egg whites
- 2 eggs
- 6 oz cream cheese
- 1 tbsp coconut or almond flour
- ½ tsp salt
- 1½ tsp ground psyllium husk powder

For filling:

- 1 tbsp oil or butter
- 5 oz cheese of your choice
- 1 oz spinach leaves

Directions

1. Preheat the oven to 400°F.
2. Beat eggs and egg whites until fluffy, then mix in cream cheese until smooth.
3. Combine salt, psyllium husk powder, and flour and mix well.
4. Fold into batter and beat. Let sit for a few minutes. The batter should look like pancake batter. Add additional psyllium husk powder if too thin.
5. Line sheet with parchment paper. Spread batter over it or make into pancakes. Bake for 5-10 minutes on the top rack.
6. Cut into six pieces. Heat oil in a skillet and fry tortilla on it. Add spinach and cheese to the center. Top with another tortilla. Fry for 1 minute on each side or until cheese melted.
7. Cut into slices and serve hot.

Nutritional Information

Servings: 6 slices
Calories: 100 per slice
Fat: 2 g
Protein: 5 g
Carbs: 10 g

Keto Grilled Cheese Sandwich

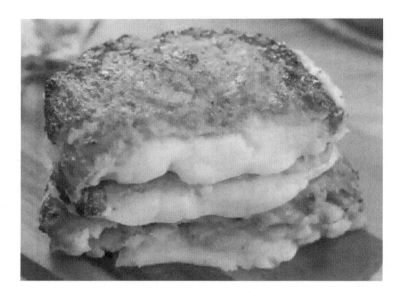

Ingredients

- 2 oz sharp cheddar cheese
- 2 large eggs, divided
- 5 tbsps butter, divided
- 4 tbsps whole milk, divided
- 1/4 tsp salt, divided
- 4 tbsps coconut flour, divided
- 1 tsp baking powder, divided

Directions

1. Place 2 tbsps butter in a container and melt in microwave.
2. Mix in milk, 1 egg, and 1/8 tsp salt. Add 2 tbsps coconut flour and ½ tsp baking powder and mix well.
3. Microwave for 90 seconds. Let cool. Slice with bread knife to make smooth like non-keto bread if desired. Repeat steps 1 to 3 to make the second portion of bread.
4. Melt butter over low heat.
5. Place cheese between bread. Place in skillet and cook until bread is golden brown, 3 minutes or so on each side. Serve hot with tomato soup.

Nutritional Information

Servings: 1 sandwich
Calories: 520 per sandwich
Fat: 46 g
Protein: 116 g
Carbs: 10 g

Stuffed Tomato Cheeseburgers

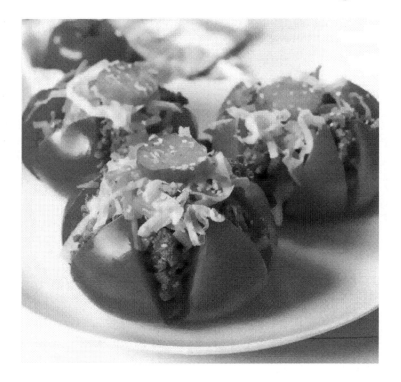

Ingredients

- 1 tbsp olive oil
- 1 medium onion, chopped
- 2 cloves garlic, minced
- 1 lb ground beef (higher fat is better!)
- 1 tbsp yellow mustard
- 4 tomatoes, sliced
- Salt and pepper to taste
- ⅔ c. cheddar cheese, shredded
- ½ c iceberg lettuce, shredded
- 4 pickles if you wish
- 1 tbsp keto ketchup (Find recipe under "Sauces")

Directions

1. Sauté onions in oil until tender, then stir in garlic. Then add ground beef and brown. Now stir in ketchup and mustard.
2. Cut tomatoes into six wedges each without breaking or separating them. Place beef mixtures between slices.
3. Top with lettuce and tomatoes and pickles if you wish.

Nutritional Information

Servings: 4
Calories: 175 per tomato
Fat: 14 g
Protein: 10 g
Carbs: 1 g

Turkey Cheese Keto Roll-Ups

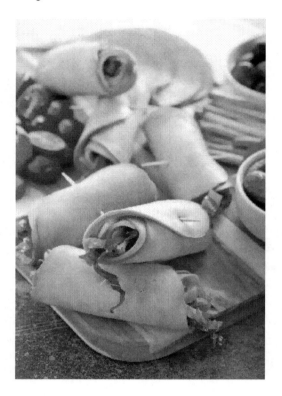

Ingredients

- 1 3-oz block of cream cheese
- 6 deli turkey slices
- black olives if you wish
- pickles if you wish
- cherry tomatoes sliced in half if desired
- 2 oz cheddar cheese, sliced

Directions

1. Spread cream cheese on turkey, place veggies inside, and roll into a tube shape.
2. Enjoy with mustard, mayo, or keto ketchup.

Nutritional Information

Servings: 6 rolls-ups
Calories: 75 per roll
Fat: 10 g
Protein: 5 g
Carbs: 0 g

Keto Stuffed Poblano Peppers

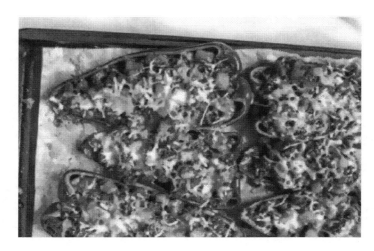

Ingredients

- 1 tbsp olive oil
- 4 poblano peppers
- 1 lb extra-lean ground beef (or ground turkey)
- 2 cloves garlic, minced
- 1 tbsp chili powder
- 1 tsp cumin
- 1 tsp paprika
- 1 red pepper, diced
- 1 red onion, diced
- 1/2 c cheddar cheese, shredded
- Pica de Gallo, sour cream, and guacamole for garnish

Directions

1. Preheat oven to 400°F. Wash and de-seed poblano peppers, then drizzle with olive oil and season with salt and pepper.
2. Bake for 10 minutes.
3. Brown the beef for about five minutes, then drain fat. Add chili powder, cumin, paprika, salt, garlic, red pepper, and red onion and sauté for 2 minutes until veggies are tender.
4. Stuff into peppers and top with cheese. Bake another 10 minutes to melt cheese.
5. Remove from oven and serve with side dish of choice.

Nutritional Information

Calories: 429
Fat: 28 g
Protein: 34 g
Carbs: 11 g

Italian Keto Roll-Ups

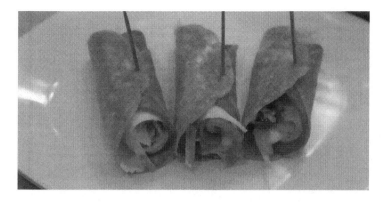

Ingredients

- 4 slices provolone cheese
- 4 slices Genoa salami
- 4 slices Mortadella
- 4 Slices Sopressata
- 4 Slices Pepperoni
- lime mayoto taste
- lettuce, ribboned or shredded to taste
- Italian seasoning to taste
- Avocado oil or olive oil (for dipping)
- Toothpicks

Directions

1. Layer meat from biggest to smallest, 1 slice per roll.
2. Spread with lime mayo.
3. Add 1 slice of cheese. Then add a few shreds of lettuce to the lower half. Then add banana peppers, jalapenos or your veggies of choice to the bottom. Sprinkle with Italian seasoning.
4. Roll up. Pin with a toothpick.
5. Serve with oil and vinegar for dipping or with keto ranch.

Nutritional Information

Calories: 243
Fat: 20 g
Protein: 10 g
Carbs: 0 g

Dinner Recipes

Oven Baked Chicken with Garlic

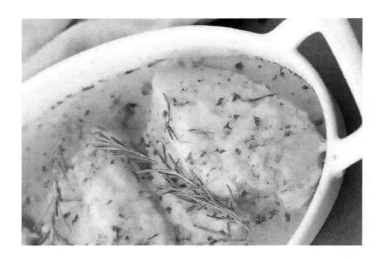

Ingredients

- 2 large chicken breasts
- ½ tsp pepper
- 2 tsp sea salt
- 1/6 stick butter
- 2 garlic cloves, minced

Directions

1. First, preheat oven to 400°F. Season chicken with salt and pepper.
2. Place chicken in a baking dish.
3. Melt butter over stove and then add garlic. Let butter cool without hardening.
4. Add garlic butter to the chicken.
5. Bake 1-1 ½ hours at 400°F. Remove from oven when internal temperature of chicken reaches at least 180°F. Baste with juices from the bottom of the pan every 20 minutes to keep moist.

Nutritional Information

Servings: 2 breasts
Calories: 197 per breast
Fat: 7. 8 g
Protein: 30 g
Carbs: 1 g

Salmon with Lemon

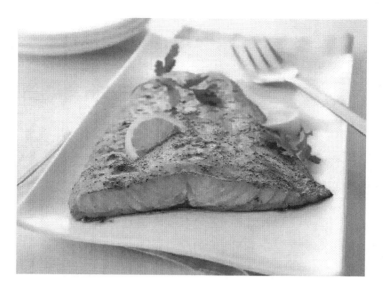

Ingredients

- 2 3-oz salmon filets
- 1 tbsp olive oil
- Ground black pepper to taste
- 1 tsp sea salt
- half stick butter
- 1 lemon, zested

Directions

1. Preheat the oven to 400°F.
2. Grease baking dish with olive oil. Lay salmon down skin side down. Add salt and pepper to taste.
3. Thinly slice lemon and place on top of salmon. Slice butter and lay thin slices on top of salmon and lemon slices.
4. Bake on middle rack for about 20–30 minutes, or until salmon is white and flakes with a fork.
5. Melt rest of butter, then let cool. Squeeze in lemon juice. Pour into a bowl and serve alongside salmon. Pairs well with asparagus.

Nutritional Information

Servings: 2 salmon filets
Calories: 170 per oz
Fat: 6 g
Protein: 26 g
Carbs: 0 g

Keto Bacon-Wrapped Meatloaf

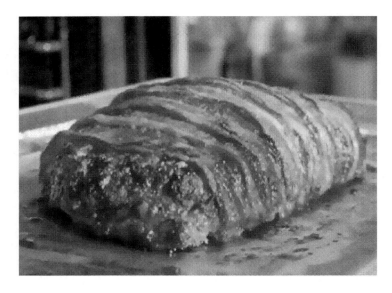

Ingredients

- 1 tbsp extra-virgin olive oil
- 1 medium onion, chopped
- 1 celery stalk, chopped
- 3 cloves garlic, minced
- 2 eggs
- 1 tsp dried oregano
- 1 tsp chili powder
- 1/2 c almond flour
- 2 lb ground beef
- Freshly ground black pepper
- 1 c cheddar cheese, shredded
- 1/4 c parmesan cheese, grated
- 1 tbsp low-sodium soy sauce
- Kosher salt
- 6 strips bacon

Directions

1. Preheat oven to 400°F. Grease a medium baking dish.
2. Heat oil over stove. Sauté onion and celery until soft. Add garlic, oregano, chili powder and cook till fragrant. Let mixture cool.
3. Mix other ingredients in a big bowl. Shape into a loaf and wrap in bacon. Place in oven.
4. Cook until bacon crispy and beef cooked. This should take about 1 hour.

Nutritional Information

Servings: 16 oz
Calories: 158 per oz
Fat: 14 g
Protein: 6 g
Carbs: 2 g

Low-Carb Lamb Sliders

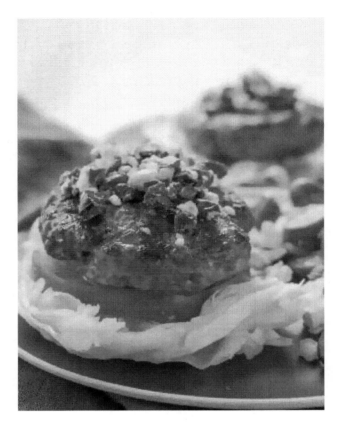

Ingredients

- 1 lb ground lamb
- 1 lemon, zested
- ½ tsp ground black pepper
- ¼ yellow onion
- 2 garlic cloves, minced
- 2 tsp fresh oregano leaves
- ½ tsp sea salt

Directions

1. Season lamb in a bowl with salt and pepper.
2. Add the diced onion, minced garlic, oregano leaves, and lemon zest. Mix until the meat is coated evenly.
3. Preheat grill to medium-high heat.
4. Form 6-8 patties.
5. Grill the burgers about 4 minutes per side over medium high heat, or until grilled through.

Nutritional Information

Servings: 6 sliders
Calories: 258 per slider
Fat: 16.5 g
Protein: 21 g
Carbs: 4 g

Keto Cuban Roast Pork

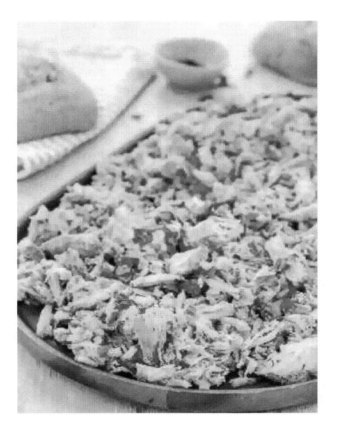

Ingredients

- 4 boneless pork shoulders
- 2 tsp ground cumin
- 4 tsp fine salt
- 1 tsp pepper
- ¼ c olive oil
- 5 sprigs fresh oregano
- 1 large red onion, diced
- 4 cloves garlic
- 1 orange, juiced
- 2 lemons, juiced

Directions

1. Rub pork shoulder with salt and place in a large bowl.
2. Combine the rest of the ingredients in a food processor and pulse until combined.
3. Pour marinade over meat and rub into it. Cover and marinate in the fridge for at least eight hours, turning over halfway.
4. Place at room temperature for 1 hour.
5. Place in the crockpot or pressure cooker, fat side up. Coat in marinade.
6. Cook on high for 40 minutes or if in a crockpot, cook on low for 8 hours.
7. Pre-heat the oven to 425°F.
8. Place the pork shoulder fat side up on a sheet pan and roast for 30 minutes or until golden and crispy.
9. Reduce the juice left behind in the pressure cooker for 20 minutes.
10. Shred the pork shoulder and pour the reduced marinade all over. Serve with riced cauliflower or zucchini chunks.

Nutritional Information

Servings: 4
Calories: 300 for 1 serving
Fat: 36 g
Protein: 14 g
Carbs: 5 g

Keto Chicken Wings

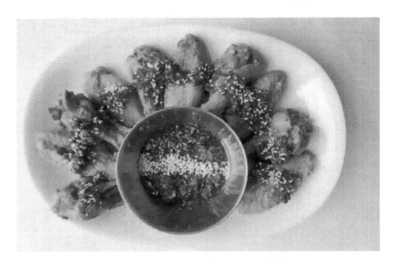

Ingredients

- 10 medium chicken wings
- 1 tbsp baking powder
- 1 tsp salt

Directions

1. Pat chicken wings with a paper towel and place on a cutting board. Sprinkle with salt on both sides and let stand for 1 hour.
2. Once again, pat chicken wings with a paper towel and place in a bag.
3. Add 1 tbsp of baking powder and 1/2 tsp of salt to the bag. Shake to evenly coat the chicken wings.
4. Bake at 250°F for 30 minutes on a greased sheet.
5. Turn the oven up to 450°F and bake for an additional 30-40 minutes or until golden and crispy.
6. Remove chicken wings from oven and cool for 5 minutes. Toss in a keto sauce of your choice and enjoy!

Nutritional Information

Servings: 10 wings
Calories: 61 per wing
Fat: 4 g
Protein: 5 g
Carbs: 0 g

Keto Bacon Cheeseburger Bake

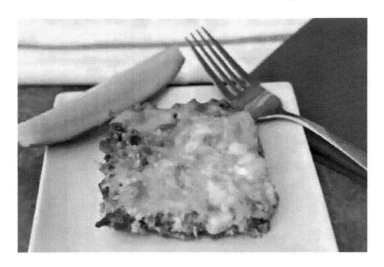

Ingredients

- 1 lb hamburger
- 1 c onion, chopped
- 2 garlic cloves, minced
- 1 tsp Worcestershire sauce
- 2 oz cream cheese
- 2 eggs
- 1-2 tbsps mustard
- 1/2 c heavy whipping cream
- 1 c cheddar cheese, shredded, divided
- 1 c white cheddar cheese, shredded, divided
- Salt and pepper to taste
- 1 tsp all seasoning
- 3 slices bacon, crumbled
- 1 kosher pickle, sliced into pieces

Directions

1. Preheat oven to 350°F.
2. In a skillet, brown hamburger with garlic, all season, onions, salt and pepper. Then add cream cheese and Worcestershire sauce and cook until cream cheese is melted.
3. Remove the skillet from the heat.
4. In a medium bowl, combine eggs, cheeses, heavy cream, and mustard.
5. Grease baking dish. Pour the ground beef mixture into the dish and add bacon and pickles.
6. Place the heavy cream mixture on top. Sprinkle remaining cheese on top.
7. Bake for 15-20 minutes or until the cheese begins to bubble.
8. Cool before serving. Add more pickles on top and lettuce and tomatoes too if you wish.

Nutritional Information

Servings: 4
Calories: 392 for 1 serving
Fat: 31 g
Protein: 27 g
Carbs: 2 g

Tuna Casserole

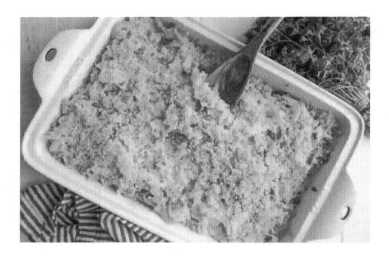

Ingredients

- 2 small cans tuna, drained
- 1/3 c mayo
- 1 tbsp Dijon mustard
- 1/4 c chopped onion
- 1/4 tsp sea salt
- 1/4 tsp pepper
- ¼ tsp cayenne pepper
- 1/2 c gruyere cheese, shredded, divided
- ¼ c parsley, chopped (optional)

Directions

1. Preheat oven to 400°F.
2. Mix together the tuna, mayonnaise, mustard, ¼ c gruyere cheese, and everything else in a bowl (reserving ¼ c gruyere cheese for later). Mix well.
3. Place in a casserole dish. Top with remaining cheese.
4. Bake for 15 minutes. Sprinkle with parsley and serve with a veggie side dish.

Nutritional Information

Servings: 3
Calories: 465 for 1 serving
Fat: 36 g
Protein: 33 g
Carbs: 2 g

Keto Stuffed Bell Peppers

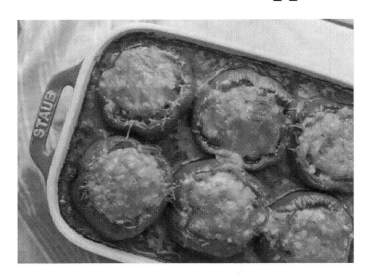

Ingredients

- 1 lb ground beef (more fat is better)
- 4 big bell peppers
- 1 tbsp olive oil
- 1/4 c keto barbecue sauce
- 2 cs cauliflower rice
- 1 tsp salt, divided
- 1/2 tsp black pepper, divided
- 1 tsp oregano
- 2 cloves garlic, pressed for juice
- 1/4 c onion, chopped
- Salt and pepper to taste

Directions

1. Preheat oven to 400°F.
2. Wash peppers and remove tops and insides. Season with salt and pepper to taste.
3. Sauté onions and garlic in olive oil until fragrant. Add beef and half of the salt and pepper, and the oregano. Cook until meat browns.
4. Add barbecue sauce and cauliflower rice and the remaining salt and pepper. Cook for 2 minutes and stir often.
5. Stuff peppers with mixture. Wrap them in foil and add tops back to peppers.
6. Bake for 1 hour at 400°F. Then take tops off and bake for another 10 minutes until soft. Add cheese on top if you wish and serve warm.

Nutritional Information

Servings: 4
Calories: 193 per pepper
Fat: 13 g
Protein: 11 g
Carbs: 6 g

Keto Pesto Salmon

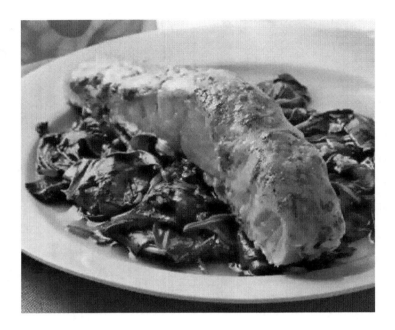

Ingredients

- 4 3-oz salmon filets
- 1 c fresh cilantro
- 3 tbsp lime juice
- Salt and pepper to taste
- 3 cloves garlic
- 2 tbsp olive oil

Directions

1. Blend garlic, olive oil, cilantro, and lime juice in a food processor to a puree. This is your pesto.
2. Add salt and pepper to your salmon filets.
3. Preheat oven to 475°F.
4. Heat olive oil over stove. Cook salmon for 5 minutes. Then throw in the oven for 3 minutes.
5. Pour pesto on top. Serve with creamed spinach, brussels sprouts, or asparagus. You can use keto hollandaise sauce instead of pesto if you wish.

Nutritional Information

Servings: 4
Calories: 227 per filet
Fat: 14 g
Protein: 22 g
Carbs: 0.1 g

Pimiento Cheese Meatballs with Zucchini Pasta

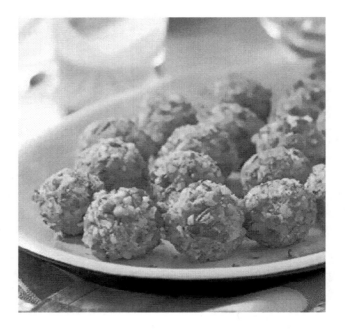

Ingredients

- zucchini noodles (make your own by spiralizing some zucchinis or buy them in stores)
- 2 oz cream cheese
- 2 c Monterey cheese
- 2 c sharp cheddar cheese
- 1 tsp onion, grated
- ⅛ tsp garlic powder
- 3 tbsps mayonnaise
- 3 tbsps pimientos, chopped, drained
- pinch salt
- pinch freshly ground pepper
- 1½ cs roasted pecans, finely chopped

Directions

1. Process cream cheese in a food processor until smooth. Then add the Monterey Jack cheese, cheddar cheese, mayonnaise, pimientos, onion, garlic powder, salt, and pepper and pulse.
2. Scrape into a bowl, cover, and refrigerate for 30 minutes to 2 days.
3. Place pecans in a medium bowl. Roll the cheese mixture into 1-inch balls and coat each ball with pecans. These are your meatballs.
4. Microwave or boil zucchini noodles until soft. Serve with meatballs.

Nutritional Information

Servings: 12 balls
Calories: 66 per ball
Fat: 6 g
Protein: 3 g
Carbs: 0 g

Roasted Turkey with Keto Cream Cheese Sauce

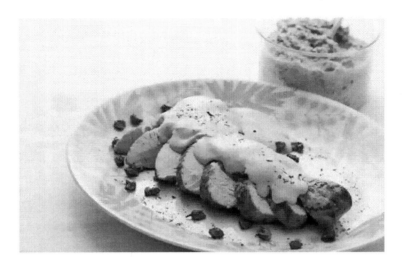

Ingredients

- 1½ lbs turkey breast
- 2 tbsp butter
- 2 cs heavy whipping cream
- 7 oz cream cheese
- Salt and pepper to taste
- ⅓ c small capers
- 1 tbsp tamari soy sauce

Directions

1. Preheat the oven to 350°F.
2. In a skillet, melt half of the butter over medium heat and then fry the turkey breast until golden brown all around.
3. Bake turkey breast in the oven. Then place on a plate, and tent with foil.
4. Pour turkey drippings into a small saucepan and add whipping cream and cream cheese. Stir and bring to a light boil. Lower the heat and simmer until thickened. Add soy sauce, salt and pepper.
5. Sauté the capers until crispy.
6. Serve turkey breast topped with sauce and fried capers.

Nutritional Information

Servings: 8
Calories: 815 per breast
Fat: 67 g
Protein: 47 g
Carbs: 7 g

Keto Crack Chicken

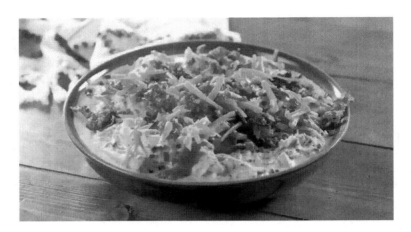

Ingredients

- 2 c. low-sodium chicken broth
- 2 lb. boneless skinless chicken breasts
- 2 tsp dill, dried
- 1 tsp chives, dried
- 1 tbsp parsley, dried
- 1/2 tsp onion powder
- 1/4 tsp garlic powder
- Kosher salt to taste
- Freshly ground black pepper to taste
- 2 (8-oz) blocks cream cheese, cubed
- 2 1/4 c. cheddar cheese, shredded
- 8 slices bacon, crumbled
- Chopped chives if you wish

Directions

1. Pour chicken broth into slow cooker and stir in dried parsley, dill, onion powder, and garlic. Add half the chicken and season with salt and pepper.
2. Repeat with remaining half of chicken. Stir to coat chicken evenly and cook on low for 6 hours or high for 2 hours.
3. Using two forks, shred chicken. Stir in cream cheese and 2 cs cheddar cheese and melt.
4. Top with remaining 1/4 c cheddar cheese, bacon, and chives.

Nutritional Information

Servings: 8 cups
Calories: 400 per cup
Fat: 40 g
Protein: 5 g
Carbs: 2 g

Keto Chicken Enchilada

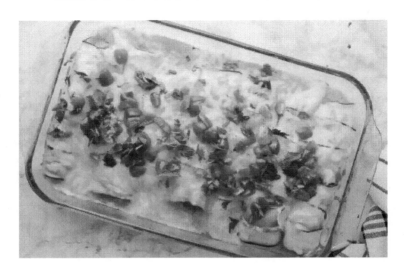

Ingredients

- 1 can Hatch green chile enchilada sauce
- 10 low carb tortillas (can make your own using cauliflower or almond flour or buy them from Mission)
- 1 c cheddar cheese, shredded
- 16 oz chicken breast or thigh meat if preferred, shredded
- 1/2 c green onions, sliced
- Cilantro, chopped

Directions

1. Allow sauce to simmer. Shred chicken, season with salt and pepper, and set aside.
2. Preheat oven to 350°F. Spoon a little sauce in the bottom of a baking pan.
3. Place a tortilla on your work surface. Put 2 tbsps of cheddar cheese in a line down the middle of the tortilla and add 1/4 c of chicken on top of the cheddar cheese.
4. Roll the tortilla up and place it down in the baking pan. Continue until you run out of ingredients.
5. Place any left-over chicken on top of the enchiladas. Pour the enchilada sauce over the enchiladas with the remaining cheddar cheese, green onions and sauce.
6. Bake for 30 minutes. Garnish with cilantro, guacamole, and sour cream.

Nutritional Information

Servings: 6
Calories: 422 for 1 serving
Fat: 30 g
Protein: 31 g
Carbs: 19 g

Ketogenic Soups

Keto Chili

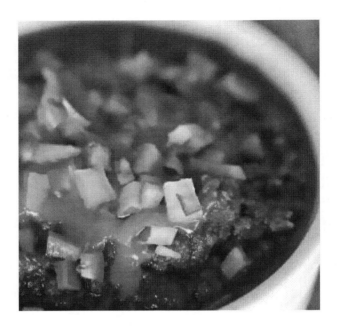

Ingredients

- 1 ½ pounds ground beef
- 2 tbsp chili powder
- 1 tsp cumin
- 1 tsp salt
- 1 yellow onion, diced
- 1 green pepper, diced
- 1 jalapeno pepper, minced
- 1 clove garlic, minced
- 2 cs beef broth
- ¼ c tomato paste
- 15 oz can diced tomatoes

Directions

1. Mix the ground beef, onion, and bell pepper in a large pan and cook over medium heat. Stir while cooks. When meat is cooked through, drain fat from pan.
2. Add the jalapeno, garlic, tomato paste, diced tomatoes, beef broth, chili powder, cumin, and salt. Stir.
3. Bring to a boil and reduce to a simmer. Simmer for at least 20 minutes.
4. Serve topped with sour cream and shredded cheddar cheese.

Nutritional Information

Servings: 6 cups
Calories: 357 per cup
Fat: 21g
Protein: 33g
Carbs: 9g

Keto Cream of Asparagus

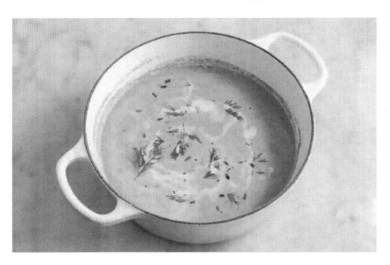

Ingredients

- 2 c vegetable stock
- 3 c butter, unsalted
- 2 tbsp asparagus, chopped
- 1½ tbsp red onion
- 1 clove garlic
- 1/3 c heavy cream
- ¼ tsp sea salt
- 1/8 black pepper

Directions

1. Heat butter and sauté garlic and onion.
2. Dice soft parts of asparagus into small pieces and fry in mixture for 4 minutes or until tender.
3. Add vegetable stock and boil. Simmer for 5-6 minutes.
4. Blend until creamy.
5. Stir with cream in pan and add salt and pepper. You can garnish with paprika or green onions.

Nutritional Information

Servings: 6 cups
Calories: 154 per cup
Fat: 14 g
Protein: 3 g
Carbs: 4 g

Keto Cauliflower Bacon Chowder

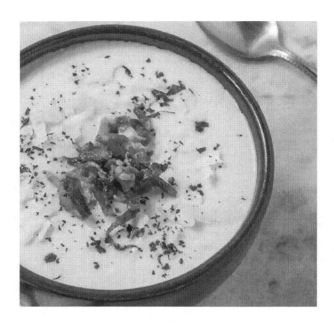

Ingredients

- 1 oz butter
- 2 cloves garlic, crushed
- 1.3 pounds (1 medium head) cauliflower, cut into evenly sized florets
- 2 cs chicken stock
- ⅔ c parmesan cheese, shaved
- 10 oz heavy cream
- 1 tsp black pepper
- 7 oz bacon
- Salt to taste

Directions

1. Melt butter and sauté garlic for 2 minutes or until soft.
2. Add cauliflower. Stir. Sauté for 2 minutes.
3. Now add heavy cream, chicken stock, black pepper and reduce to a simmer for 20 minutes.
4. While the cauliflower is cooking, fry the bacon and cut it into thin slices.
5. Mix the bacon and soup together in a blender and purée.
6. Add parmesan cheese and stir. Add salt if you wish.

Nutritional Information

Servings: 6 cups
Calories 421 per cup
Fat 38 g
Protein: 13 g
Carbs 7g

Keto Thai Curry Soup

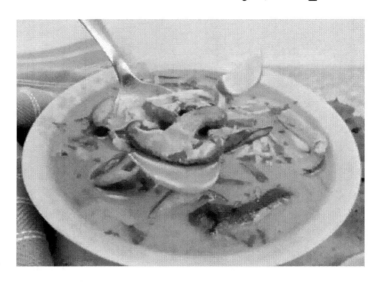

Ingredients

- 4 chicken breasts
- 14 oz chicken broth
- 28 oz water
- 14 oz coconut milk
- 2 tbsps Thai garlic chili sauce
- 1 tbsp coconut aminos
- 1 tsp ginger, ground
- 1 oz lime juice
- 2 sprigs basil
- Cilantro, chopped

Directions

1. Thinly slice the chicken breast then cut them up into bite-sized pieces.
2. In a large pot, combine coconut milk, broth, water, chili sauce, coconut aminos, lime juice, ginger, and basil. Boil over high heat.
3. Add chicken pieces, reduce heat to low-medium, and cover. Simmer for 30 minutes.
4. Fish out basil leaves from the soup and garnish with cilantro.

Nutritional Information

Servings: 10 cups
Calories: 227 per cup
Fat: 16 g
Protein: 18 g
Carbs: 3 g

Keto Cream of Zucchini

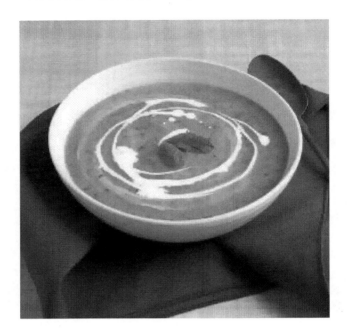

Ingredients

- 1 medium onion, chopped
- 1 tbsp butter
- 1/2 tsp sea salt
- 4 medium zucchini
- 4 cs vegetable broth
- 1/2 c heavy cream
- Freshly ground nutmeg

Directions

1. Heat a medium pot over medium-high heat and melt butter. Add onion and salt. Stir until onion is translucent.
2. Chop zucchini. Add zucchini and broth to the onion. Boil then simmer for 15 minutes or when zucchini is tender.
3. Blend soup to a fine puree.
4. Return the pureed soup to the pot.
5. Stir in cream and heat over low heat.
6. Add salt and pepper to taste. Serve hot with a sprinkle of nutmeg or paprika.

Nutritional Information

Servings: 5 cups
Calories: 130 per cup
Fat: 10 g
Protein: 4 g
Carbs: 3 g

Ketogenic Desserts
Coconut Macadamia Bars

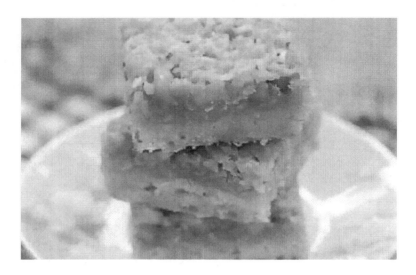

Ingredients

For the Crust:

- 1 1/4 c almond flour, coconut flour or some flour alternative
- 1/3 c sugar-free liquid sweetener
- 1/4 tsp salt
- 1/4 c butter chilled, chopped into small bits

For the Filling:

- 1/4 c butter
- 1/2 c sugar-free liquid sweetener
- 1/2 c coconut cream
- 1 1/3 c coconut flakes
- 3/4 c macadamia nuts, chopped
- 1 egg yolk
- 1/2 tsp vanilla extract

Directions

For the Crust:

1. First preheat the oven to 350°F. Mix flour, sweetener, and salt and pulse in a food processor. Add butter and keep pulsing into fine chunks.
2. Press into pan and bake for 15 minutes. Then let cool.

For the Filling:

1. Melt butter. Then add in coconut cream and sugar-free liquid sweetener, and whisk till smooth.
2. Now add coconut flakes, macadamia nuts, egg yolk, and vanilla extract and stir well. Add to crust.
3. Bake for 40 minutes or until edges brown. Let cool to set the soft center and then cut into bars.

Nutritional Information

Servings: 8 bars
Calories: 199 per bar
Fat: 19.3 g
Protein: 3.1 g
Carbs: 4.3 g

Almond Butter Pie

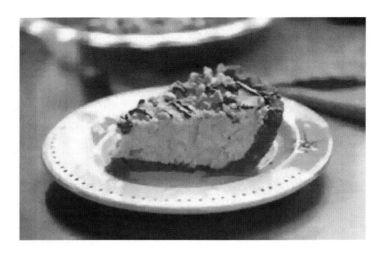

Ingredients

- Any type of low-carb pie crust 6" size
- 3/4 c almond milk
- 1/2 c heavy cream
- 1/2 c granulated sweetener sugar-free
- 1 tbsp cornstarch
- 4 eggs
- ¼ tsp xanthan gum
- 2 tsps vanilla extract
- 1/4 tsp salt
- 2/3 c peanut butter or any nut butter of your choice
- 1/2 c heavy cream
- 2 tbsps icing sugar

Whipped Cream Topping

- 1 c heavy cream
- 1/4 c icing sugar

Directions

1. Pour almond milk and heavy cream into a medium sauce pan over medium heat and heat until milk simmers.
2. Stir dry ingredients in a bowl and then add eggs and mix well.
3. Slowly add hot milk and cream into egg mixture and whisk. Put pudding back on stove and scrape pudding out. Place sieve over the empty mixing bowl.
4. Turn the heat to medium and begin whisking the pudding mixture. It will thicken and look grainy after about 5 minutes. Turn heat down, whisk for another minute. Take off heat and whisk some more.
5. Pour/scrape the pudding into the sieve to strain out any egg or lumps. Add the vanilla to the pudding and stir. Add the peanut butter to the pudding and stir. Taste for seasoning. Add powdered sweetener to make sweeter if you wish. Add more salt if you wish. Put a piece of plastic wrap over the pudding and let cool completely in the fridge.
6. Now measure ½ c heavy cream into a bowl. Add sweetener and 2 pinches xanthan gum. Whip until stiff. Add to pudding, folding until white is gone.
7. Pour the remaining heavy cream into bowl and add sweetener and 1/8 tsp gum. Whip until creamy but not stiff. Set aside; this is your topping.
8. Now add pudding to crust. Top with topping. You can add shaved dark chocolate or nuts on top. Serve chilled the next day.

Nutritional Information

Servings: 6
Calories: 472 per slice (1/6 of pie)
Fat: 44 g
Protein: 14 g
Carbs: 8 g

Flourless Chocolate Brownies

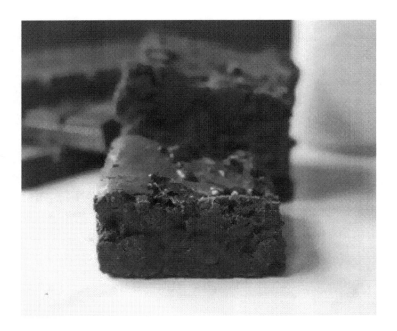

Ingredients

- 12 tbsp butter, unsalted
- 1/2 tsp salt
- 1 1/2 cs sugar, granulated
- 2 tsp coffee or vanilla extract
- 2 cs milk chocolate chips or chopped milk chocolate
- 4 eggs
- 2 tbsp cocoa powder, unsweetened
- 6 tbsp cornstarch

Directions

1. Preheat oven to 350°F.
2. Line square baking pan with foil and butter or oil.
3. Melt butter. Whisk in sugar. Add chocolate chips and stir till melted.
4. Take off stove and let cool before adding eggs and coffee/vanilla extract.
5. Using a sifter, sift cocoa powder and cornstarch into the saucepan, then add salt. Whisk till smoothPour batter into a pan.
6. Bake for 22-28 minutes. Jiggle brownies to see if they're done.
7. Let cool for 45 minutes before cutting into squares.

Nutritional Information

Servings: 6
Calories: 43 per brownie
Fat: .3 g
Protein: 1.5 g
Carbs: 8.9 g

No-Bake Peanut Butter Chocolate Bars

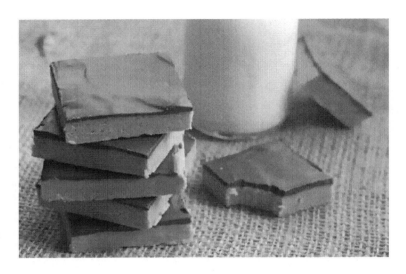

Ingredients

For the Bars:

- 3/4 c almond flour
- 2 oz butter
- ¼ c icing sugar
- ½ c peanut butter
- Vanilla extract to taste

For the Topping:

- 1/2 c chocolate chips

Directions

1. Mix all the ingredients for the bars together and spread into a small pan.
2. Melt the chocolate chips in a microwave oven for 30 seconds and stir till smooth.
3. Spread chocolate on top of the batter for the bars.
4. Chill for at least 2 hours to thicken before serving.

Nutritional Information

Servings: 12
Calories: 246 per bar
Fat: 23 g
Protein: 7 g
Carbs: 7 g

Keto Peppermint Bars

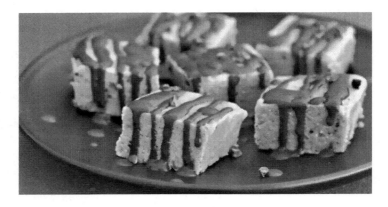

Ingredients

For the Base:

- 1 c almond flour
- 1/2 c butter
- 1 c chocolate chips

For the Topping:

- 1/3 c powdered sweetener
- 1 tsp peppermint extract
- 1/4 c butter, softened
- 6 tbsps heavy cream
- 1 drop green food coloring (optional)

Directions

1. Lightly grease 8 x 6 inch square pan.
2. Melt butter and chocolate in microwave and stir well. Add in flour. Mix well then set in fridge.
3. Beat ¼ c butter, cream, peppermint, and food coloring and mix until smooth. Beat in powdered sweetener until smooth.
4. Smooth over top of bars.
5. Chill for 15-20 minutes in fridge.
6. Cut into bars and drizzle any leftover chocolate/butter on top.

Nutritional Information

Servings: 12
Calories: 215 per bar
Fat: 21 g
Protein: 3 g
Carbs: 8 g

Keto Carrot Cake

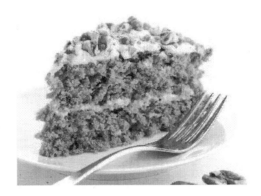

Ingredients

For the icing:

- 8 oz cream cheese softened in microwave for 10 seconds
- 1/2 c butter, softened
- 1/2 c powdered erythritol
- 1 tsp vanilla extract
- 2 tbsp heavy cream

For the carrot cake:

- 5 eggs
- 3/4 c erythritol
- 1 1/4 c carrot, shredded
- 2 tsp vanilla extract
- 14 tbsp butter, melted
- 1/4 c coconut, shredded
- 1/4 tsp salt
- 1 3/4 c almond flour
- 1/2 c coconut flour
- 2 tsp baking powder
- 1 1/2 tsp cinnamon, ground

Directions

For the icing:

1. Beat cream cheese and butter. Add sweetener and beat more.
2. Add vanilla extract and heavy cream and beat. Fold in more heavy cream until it gets to be thick.
3. Preheat oven to 350°F. Line the bottoms of two 8-inch cake pans with parchment paper and grease.
4. Beat eggs and erythritol for 5 minutes on medium-high till fluffy. Then add vanilla.

For the carrot cake:

1. Sift dry ingredients in bowl. Fold into egg mixture.
2. Add the coconut and stir to combine. Add carrots. Add melted butter. Mix well.
3. Divide the batter between pans. Bake for 30 minutes or until toothpick comes out clean.
4. Let the cakes cool inside the pans for 10-15 minutes. Cut into large even parts once cool.
5. Place cake layer on platter, spread icing, then add second layer, and spread more frosting. Frost sides.
6. Chill for 30 minutes.

Nutritional Information

Servings: 6 slices
Calories: 307 per slice
Fat: 29 g
Protein: 6 g
Carbs: 7 g

Keto No-Bake Coconut Peanut Butter Cookies

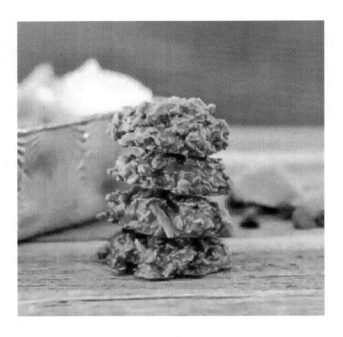

Ingredients

- 1 1/3 cs creamy peanut butter
- 1 tsp erythritol (optional)
- 2 tsps vanilla extract
- 2 tbsps cocoa powder, unsweetened
- 2 cs coconut flakes, unsweetened
- 2 tbsps butter, melted

Directions

1. Line baking sheet with parchment paper.
2. Combine peanut butter, vanilla, melted butter, coconut flakes, and cocoa powder and stir well.
3. Prepare a large baking sheet with parchment paper or a non-stick silicone baking mat.
4. Scoop batter onto sheet. Press into cookie shapes with spoon.
5. Freeze for 30 minutes.

Nutritional Information

Servings: 12 cookies
Calories: 153 for two cookies
Fat: 13 g
Protein: 4 g
Carbs: 5 g

Carb-Free Raspberry Dream Cheesecake

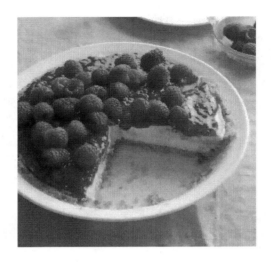

Ingredients

For the crust:

- 2 cs almond flour
- 1/3 c butter, melted
- 3 tbsps powdered sweetener
- 1 tsp vanilla

For the filling:

- 4 3-oz packages cream cheese, softened
- 1.5 c sweetener, powdered
- 4 eggs
- 1 tbsp lemon juice
- ¼ tbsp lemon zest
- 1 tsp vanilla extract
- 1 c fresh raspberries
- 2 tbsps powdered sweetener

Directions

1. Preheat the oven to 350°F. Grease spring-form pan with butter and line with parchment paper.
2. Combine almond flour, butter, sweetener, and vanilla extract in food processor and make large sticky crumbs. Press into spring-form pan to make crust. Bake for about 10 minutes and allow to cool.
3. Reduce oven temperature to 325°F.
4. Mix cream cheese and sweetener in the bowl of a mixer. Beat until smooth and combined. Add eggs one at a time while mixer is running until batter-like consistency is reached. Add lemon juice, lemon zest, and 1 tsp vanilla.
5. Add batter to crust. Smooth top. Wrap pan in foil.
6. Combine raspberries and 2 tbsps sweetener in mixer and make into a puree. Set aside some raspberries for garnish later. Fold into batter in pan.
7. Bake 75 for minutes or until firm.
8. Cool. Then lift from pan. Top with remaining puree and fresh raspberries.

Nutritional Information

Servings: 6 slices
Calories: 460 per slice
Fat: 43. 2 g
Protein: 0 g
Carbs: 32.8 g

Keto Chocolate Mug Cake

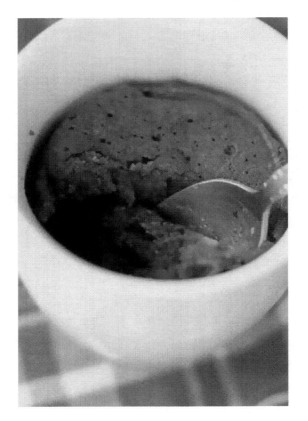

Ingredients

- 2 tbsps butter
- 1 tbsp coconut oil
- 2 tsps cocoa powder, unsweetened
- 3 tbsps almond flour
- 3 tsps erythritol
- 1 egg

Directions

1. Add butter and coconut oil to a mug. Heat till melted and stir.
2. Add all dry ingredients. Whisk well.
3. Cook for 90 minutes.

Nutritional Information

Servings: 1
Calories: 507 whole mug
Fat: 51 g
Protein: 10 g
Carbs: 6 g

Salted Caramel Cake Bombs

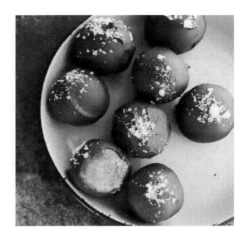

Ingredients

For the Cake:
- 2.75 cs almond flour
- 1.25 cs confectioner's sugar
- 0.5 c cocoa powder, unsweetened
- 2 tsp gluten-free baking powder
- 1/2 tsp salt
- 6 large eggs
- 1/2 c butter, melted
- 1 c pumpkin puree
- 1 tbsp vanilla extract

For the Caramel:
- 1/2 c heavy cream
- 1/2 c butter, unsalted
- 1/2 c Swerve brown sugar substitute
- 1 tsp vanilla extract
- pinch salt

For the Glaze:
- 9 oz sugar free chocolate chips
- 1 tbsp coconut oil
- Flaky sea salt

Directions

1. Preheat the oven to 325° F and line a small cake pan with parchment.
2. Beat together all cake ingredients till smooth. Bake for 55 minutes in pan.
3. Now make the caramel by combining all the ingredients for caramel in a pot over medium low heat until it starts to simmer. Simmer for 5-6 minutes. Cool.
4. Take out cake, cool, and crumble into small pieces. Pour caramel on top and mix together. Form into tiny balls and place on parchment paper and freeze.
5. Now mix chips and coconut oil and melt in microwave. Dip the balls into it. Sprinkle flaky sea salt on top. Freeze for 10 minutes before serving.

Nutritional Information

Servings: 12
Calories: 145 per bomb
Fat: 13 g
Protein: 4 g
Carbs: 4 g

Chocolate Blueberry Clusters Keto

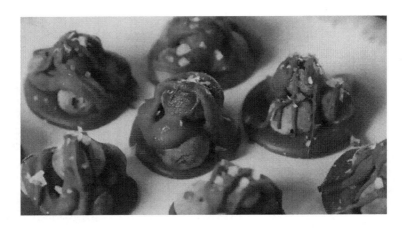

Ingredients

- 1 1/2 c. melted semisweet chocolate chips
- 1 tbsp coconut oil
- 2 c. blueberries (4 per cluster)
- Flaky sea salt

Directions

1. Line sheet with parchment paper.
2. Melt chocolate with coconut oil.
3. Spoon small amount of chocolate and top with 4 blueberries. Add a little chocolate on top.
4. Freeze for 10 minutes or until set. Top each cluster with flaky sea salt.

Nutritional Information

Servings: 15
Calories: 90 per cluster
Fat: 8 g
Protein: 0 g
Carbs: 14 g

Keto Lemon Bars

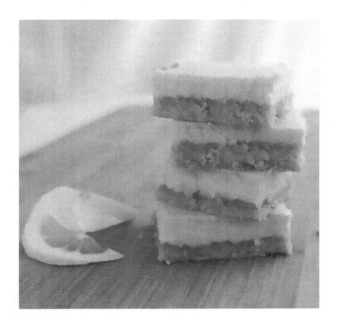

Ingredients

- 1/2 c butter, melted
- 1 3/4 cs almond flour, divided in half
- 1 c powdered erythritol, divided in half
- 3 medium lemons
- 3 eggs

Directions

1. Mix butter, 1 c almond flour, 1/4 c erythritol, and a pinch of salt. Then press on to a parchment-lined pan and bake for 20 minutes at 350°F. Let cool.
2. Mix the eggs, 3/4 c erythritol, 3/4 c almond flour, and salt.
3. Pour the filling onto the crust. Bake for 25 minutes at 350°F.
4. Chill in freezer for 20 minutes. Serve with fresh lemon slices. Can top with a sprinkle of powdered sweetener.

Nutritional Information

Servings: 6
Calories: 272
Fat: 26 g
Protein: 8 g
Carbs: 4 g

Ketogenic Sauces & Dressings

Keto Ranch

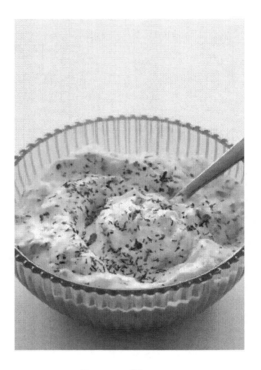

Ingredients

- 1/2 c mayonnaise
- 1/4 c heavy cream
- 1/2 c sour cream
- 2 tbsps white distilled vinegar
- 2 tbsps dill
- 2 cloves garlic, minced
- 1 tbsp parsley
- 1 tsp chives
- 1 tsp onion powder
- 1 tsp salt

Directions

1. Add all of the ingredients to a small bowl and whisk well.
2. Transfer mixture to a mason jar for storage. Store in the refrigerator for up to 5 days.

Nutritional Information

Calories in 1 tsp: 15
Fat: 3 g
Protein: 0 g
Carbs: 0 g

Keto Honey Mustard

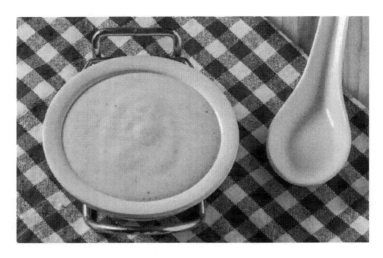

Ingredients

- 1 tbsp apple cider vinegar
- 1 tbsp yellow mustard
- 2 tsps Dijon mustard
- 1 tsp garlic powder
- 1/2 tsp paprika
- 18 drops stevia or some liquid sugar-free sweetener
- ½ c mayonnaise

Directions

1. Mix all of the ingredients together in a small bowl.
2. Refrigerate for 2 hours and serve cold.

Nutritional Information

Servings: 10
Calories: 132
Fat: 14 g
Protein: 0.2 g
Carbs: 0.7 g

Keto Ketchup

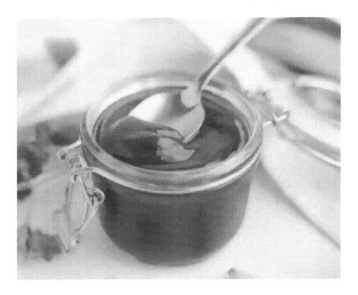

Ingredients

- 1 tomato pasta can
- 1 c water
- 1 tbsp apple cider vinegar
- 1 packet low-carb sweetener
- 1 tsp salt
- 1/2 tsp paprika
- 1 tsp garlic powder
- 1 tsp onion powder
- ½ tsp cloves

Directions

1. In a medium saucepan combine the water, tomato paste, vinegar, sweetener, garlic powder, paprika and onion powder.
2. Bring to a boil, then cover and simmer for 20-25 minutes, or until thick.
3. Add spices and salt to adjust taste.
4. Store for up to 10 days in fridge.

Nutritional Information

Servings: 14
Calories: 14
Fat: 0
Protein: 0
Carbs: 2 g

Keto Hollandaise

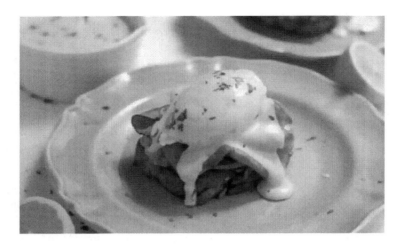

Ingredients

- 4 egg yolks
- 10 oz butter
- 2 tbsp lemon juice
- Salt and pepper to taste

Directions

1. Crack the eggs and place the egg yolks in a glass bowl.
2. Melt the butter in a sauce pan.
3. Add the butter, drop by drop, into the egg yolks while whisking. As the sauce thickens, gradually increase the amount of butter added.
4. Continue to whisk until all the butter has been added. Don't scrape the bottom of the pan used to melt the butter.
5. Add lemon juice and salt and pepper to taste. Serve immediately.

Nutritional Information

Calories: 78
Fat: 7 g
Protein: 3 g
Carbs: 0 g

Keto BBQ Sauce

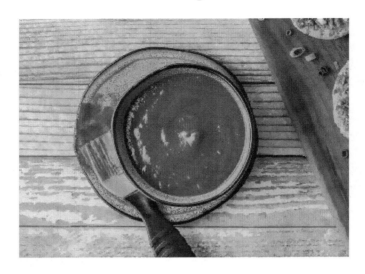

Ingredients

- 16 oz tomato sauce
- 1/4 tsps stevia, powdered
- 4 tbsps apple cider vinegar
- 4 tbsps worcestershire sauce
- 4 tsps liquid smoke flavor
- 2 tsps salt
- 2 tsps onion powder
- 1/2 tsp cayenne pepper, optional
- 1 tsp garlic, crushed

Directions

1. Place all ingredients in a saucepan.
2. Lightly simmer for 5 minutes
3. Allow to cool. Place in a jar and store in the fridge.

Nutritional Information

Calories: 9
Fat: 0 g
Protein: 0 g
Carbs: 2 g

21-DAY KETO MEAL PLAN

Day 1

Breakfast: Keto Morning Pizza

Lunch: Keto Cream of Asparagus Soup

Dinner: Grilled steak or chicken with Keto BBQ sauce

Dessert/Snack: Coconut Macadamia Bars

Day 2

Breakfast: Keto Oatmeal

Lunch: Cauliflower Nachos

Dinner: Keto Crack Chicken

Dessert/Snack: Salted Caramel Cake Bombs

Day 3

Breakfast: Keto Yummy Omelet

Lunch: Bacon Sushi

Dinner: Keto Chicken Wings with Keto Ranch

Dessert/Snack: Flourless Chocolate Brownies

Day 4

Breakfast: Omelet Bell Peppers

Lunch: Keto Thai Curry Soup

Dinner: Keto Bacon Cheeseburger Bake

Dessert/Snack: Keto Peppermint Bars

Day 5

Breakfast: Keto Muffins

Lunch: Taco Stuffed Avocados

Dinner: Keto Chicken Enchilada

Dessert/Snack: Keto Lemon Bars

Day 6

Breakfast: Nutty Creamy Pancakes

Lunch: Zucchini Pasta Salad

Dinner: Keto Crack Chicken

Dessert/Snack: Almond Butter Pie

Day 7

Breakfast: Sweet Potato with a Poached Egg

Lunch: Keto Grilled Cheese Sandwich

Dinner: Tuna Casserole

Dessert/Snack: Keto No-Bake Coconut Peanut Butter Cookies

Day 8

Breakfast: Keto Breakfast Chia Pudding

Lunch: Zucchini Pasta Salad

Dinner: Oven Baked Chicken with Garlic

Dessert/Snack: Carb-Free Raspberry Dream Cheesecake

Day 9

Breakfast: Keto Spicy Yam Breakfast Scramble

Lunch: Turkey Cheese Keto Roll-Ups

Dinner: Keto Chili

Dessert/Snack: Keto Carrot Cake

Day 10

Breakfast: Keto Waffles

Lunch: Keto Shrimp Lettuce Wraps

Dinner: Grilled Chicken, carrot sticks dipped in keto ketchup

Dessert/Snack: Keto Chocolate Mug Cake

Day 11

Breakfast: Poached Eggs with Keto Hollandaise Sauce on top

Lunch: Keto Quesadilla

Dinner: Lamb Sliders

Dessert/Snack: Keto No-Bake Coconut Peanut Butter Cookies

Day 12

Breakfast: Mushroom and Feta Keto Quiche

Lunch: Keto Cauliflower Bacon Chowder

Dinner: Roasted Turkey with Keto Cream Cheese Sauce

Dessert/Snack: Coconut Macadamia Bars

Day 13

Breakfast: Keto Cauliflower and Meat Breakfast Skillet

Lunch: Keto Cheeseburger Bake

Dinner: Salmon with Lemon

Dessert/Snack: Keto Carrot Cake

Day 14

Breakfast: Keto Breakfast Bake Breakfast Bake

Lunch: Cauliflower Nachos

Dinner: Keto Cuban Roast Pork

Dessert/Snack: Flourless Chocolate Brownies

Day 15

Breakfast: Keto Breakfast Burrito

Lunch: Italian Keto Roll-Ups

Dinner: Keto Stuffed Bell Peppers

Dessert/Snack: Salted Caramel Cake Bombs

Day 16

Breakfast: Keto Sausage and Pepper Breakfast Casserole

Lunch: Salmon Wrapped with Prosciutto

Dinner: Keto Cuban Roast Pork

Dessert/Snack: No-Bake Peanut Butter Chocolate Bars

Day 17

Breakfast: Cauliflower Cheddar Fritters

Lunch: Stuffed Tomato Cheeseburgers

Dinner: Pimiento Cheese Meatballs with Zucchini Pasta

Dessert/Snack: Keto Muffins

Day 18

Breakfast: Keto Cinnamon Rolls

Lunch: Keto Stuffed Poblano Peppers

Dinner: Keto Bacon-Wrapped Meatloaf

Dessert/Snack: Chocolate Blueberry Clusters

Day 19

Breakfast: Keto Muffins

Lunch: Keto Cream of Zucchini Soup

Dinner: Keto Pesto Salmon

Dessert/Snack: Keto Lemon Bars

Day 20

Breakfast: Baked Eggs in an Avocado

Lunch: Burger Bombs

Dinner: Tuna Casserole

Dessert/Snack: Keto Peppermint Bars

Day 21

Breakfast: Omelet Bell Peppers

Lunch: Keto Egg and Cucumber Salad

Dinner: Salmon with Lemon

Dessert/Snack: Carb-Free Raspberry Cheesecake

Manufactured by Amazon.ca
Bolton, ON